THE EATING MAN'S DIET

THE EATING MAN'S DIET

BY THOMAS SHARKEY

GROSSET & DUNLAP
A NATIONAL GENERAL COMPANY
Publishers · New York

A Castle Books, Inc. Edition
Distributed To The Trade
By Book Sales, Inc.

For My Darling Wife Felicia
—And the Magnificent Seven
(Peggy, Tommy, Martin, Mary Jane,
Maureen, Matthew and Michael)

Contents

About the Author   ix
Introduction   xi

1 Is the Eating Man's Diet for You?   1
2 The "Gimmick" Diets: Why They Work—
   Why They Don't   3
3 The "No-Gimmick" Diets: Why They Work—
   Why They Don't   8
4 The Twin Goals of Weight Reduction: Why
   Reducing Is Never Enough   14
5 You Are Not a "Foodaholic" and Should
   Never Be Treated Like One   19
6 The Search for a Better Diet—A Physical Clue   22
7 The Search for a Better Diet—
   The Psychological Key   29
8 The Secret—At Last   32
9 The Brief History of a Successful Diet   36
10 Some of the Reasons Why   43
11 Your Own Diet—Custom-Made   52
12 Some Additional Questions   60
13 Other Considerations   70
14 The Pause Before the Plunge: Are You Ready?   80

Appendix:
   Your Ideal Weight   88
   Recommended Calorie Consumption   89
   Your Daily Weight Record   90
   Comparison Calorie Counter   91
   A Guide to Your Nutritional "Musts"   114
   Eating Man's Diet Menus   115

About the Author

Thomas Sharkey weighed 10½ pounds at birth and has been dieting—and writing—most of his life.

He published his first essay at the age of 12—its subject: food. (The question was: Should We Help Feed a Starving Europe? His answer: *yes*.) It won first prize in a national contest for school children and launched his career.

Having edited and published his grammar school's first ("and probably last") newspaper, he graduated at the top of his class, a "cherub-cheeked," 5'3" 155-pounder, and spent his high school years studying for the priesthood at Chicago's Quigley Preparatory Seminary (achieving the scholastic rank of *summa cum laude*) before deciding once and for all on the writing life.

Entering DePaul University at 18 ("My weight then varied between 190 and 220 pounds—much too much for my 5'10" frame") he devoted himself to journalistic pursuits, writing a weekly column for a neighborhood newspaper, another weekly column for the school paper, editing and publishing his fraternity monthly, and helping edit both the literary quarterly and yearbook. By the time he was 21 he'd spent a year—nights—as a police reporter, had completed his first novel, acquired a literary agent, held the position of corresponding editor for the old *Chicago* Magazine and was elected president of his class.

Despite all the activity, both then and during the wealth of writing and editing jobs he's held since (his material has appeared in such diverse publications as *Home and Highway*, *Spirits* and *Reader's Digest*), his weight remained a constant problem.

It wasn't until he was 33, in fact, settled down with his wife and seven children in a small suburb 20 minutes from downtown Chicago, that he happened upon a remark made by the dean of American psychologists, William James, which was to "radically change almost every conception" he'd had about dieting.

"In that instant," he says, "I immediately saw why—despite doctors, despite pills, despite a lifetime of trying—I had continually failed to lose weight—and why, indeed, most dieters were unable to. They—and I—were attempting diets that were so designed as to *preclude the possibility of habit being formed.*"

Having devised his new, revolutionary method of combining reducing with the formation of lasting eating habits, he found, to his great surprise, that he lost 10 pounds in the first five days—and 61 pounds in six months and two days—his weight falling from a "badly overextended" 230 pounds to a "really rather trim" 169. Today, thoroughly enjoying the "wonderful world of thin," he weighs in at 160 and eats "pretty darn much" as he pleases.

Introduction

I hadn't seen my friend in a few months and as we sat down to order lunch he expressed amazement at the change in my appearance. When we'd last met I was a puffy, obese 230 pounds; I was now 59 pounds lighter—feeling and, he said, *looking* on top of the world..

What further amazed him was that he knew I'd been pursuing this goal most of my 33 years. No diet had ever made much difference. I weighed 10½ pounds at birth and sometimes it seemed I'd remain overweight until I died.

Before I could attempt to answer his question as to how I'd done it, the waitress came and we ordered. He said he'd been doing a little calorie-counting himself lately and asked for a salad, a small lean steak and black coffee. I asked for the same—*plus* a bowl of chowder, stringbeans, a baked potato, rolls and butter, and—for dessert—the deep dish apple pie a la mode.

He said, "Oh, now that it's over, you're letting down a little, is that it?"

"As a matter of fact, no." I couldn't help grinning as I answered; I'd been asked that question several times recently. "You see, I'm still *on* the diet. I've a couple of pounds to go."*

He looked bewildered. "What's the secret? Skip breakfast?"

"Not at all. For breakfast this morning I had ham and eggs—the way I like them—with provolone cheese and a little

---

* I didn't know it then of course, but I was to drop *an additional nine pounds* in the six weeks that followed the actual diet—for a total loss of 70 pounds.

jelly. I had fried potatoes on the side, a couple of pieces of toast—liberally spread with margarine and honey. Also a half-grapefruit, a glass of tomato juice and—yes—cereal with milk and sugar.

"Tonight for supper," I went on before he could protest, "I'll have a meal pretty much like this one—only I may have a martini *before* and skip the dessert *after*. Before bed I'll probably have a Scotch or two."

"Uh—how long have you been doing this?," he asked, clearly mystified.

"I began just under six months ago . . . and *I've been losing at the regular rate of 10 pounds a month.*"

The waitress arrived with my rolls. He sent her back to get some for himself and told me I'd better start explaining.

Naturally I didn't—I couldn't—give him all the details at that one sitting. Not that the diet itself was so very complicated. It wasn't. But I knew that every answer I gave was bound to inspire at least two additional questions. And, being neither a nutritionist nor a psychologist—except in the strictly nonprofessional sense—I realized all too well that I didn't have the additional answers. Not then.

How, for instance, could I have responded if he'd asked me to back up my contention that losing weight is primarily a psychological rather than a physical problem—and it must therefore be solved with psychological means?

Suppose he had requested scientific evidence for my conviction that "will power" as such has very little to do with remaining faithful to a diet—and that the overweight have, in fact, *a good deal more will power when it comes to abstaining from food* than the thin?

What would I have said if he'd demanded nutritional support for my conclusion that foods containing a high quantity of so-called "empty calories" (ice cream, beer, pizza, candy: those which are sternly ruled off most diet lists) were *absolutely essential*—assuming normal health—to the dieter who was determined to achieve and sustain his ideal weight?

Or what if he had challenged the diet's psychological principle itself and dared me to produce corroborative testimony from experts in the field?

No, I didn't have the answers then.

I knew that the diet worked. And I knew that it was

based on the strongest psychological principle known to man—a force which the Duke of Wellington once described as "ten times nature."

But it was only after many months of research—months of correspondence, personal interviews and long distance telephone conversations with physicians, nutritionists, psychiatrists and psychologists in this country and abroad—months of reading, experimenting and having my diet tested under doctor's auspices upon a wide variety of subjects—months of witnessing it being undertaken by people whose weight problems were far different from mine (some of whom had never successfully completed a diet before, and at least one who had never even *attempted* to lose weight!) and then seeing them succeed, time and again, often beyond their wildest dreams—that the answers, and this book, began to take shape.

Yes, the diet really worked all right. It worked to a degree approaching 100 per cent success (see Chapter One: *Is the Eating Man's Diet for You?*). And, as I'd suspected, there were solid, well-established scientific principles behind its every phase.

Perhaps, however, the really best part of it—and that which most distinguishes it from other diets—is not in its *ability* to work (open any diet book and you'll be promised Complete Success "if only" you'll *do* such-and-such, *eat* such-and-such, or *not eat* such-and-such) but the fact that, psychologically oriented as it is, *it turns that ability into a reality.*

That's right.

The Eating Man's Diet, once you decide to begin it, is so designed as to *seem to actually take over,* to act almost as if with an independent will of its own, continually and steadily slimming you to your ideal weight—and then helping keep you at that ideal weight for a lifetime.

It is so designed that at the very time when other diets—however generous or well-planned—begin to become most difficult, to really pall, to make you ready to climb the walls or swap your soul for an old-fashioned hot fudge sundae, the Eating Man's Diet really comes into its own.

It is at this point that, amost without your being aware of it, the "take over" begins, that *the diet becomes easier to continue than to quit,* that *you become,* in a word, willingly, happily *"hooked."*

It is at this point on the Eating Man's Diet that you begin to enjoy your food as never before—that you discover the wonder of being able to munch a handful of candy with neither a guilty conscience nor the desire to devour the entire box.

It is at this point that you find yourself willingly rising early enough in the morning to consume a big breakfast—or, if not so big a breakfast, enjoying coffee and rolls (again with no guilty conscience) along with the gang down at work.

It is at this point that you begin to fully appreciate the *joys* of a high-calorie dessert, a glass of wine, a box of buttered popcorn or simply a cup of well-creamed coffee—without the nagging desire that is all too common among the overweight to swallow it down whole, to get it into your system (and therefore "out of your system") as quickly and painlessly as possible, eating more in punishment than in pleasure.

And all the while, as you delight in these gustatory pleasures, you witness the steady, steady dropping away of pounds and inches.

Indeed, it is at this point that, perhaps for the first time, you fully realize that *you are not so different* from other, so-called "normal" eaters—that the excuses you gave yourself in the past for overeating, whether based on heredity, an over-indulgent mother, an out-of-whack appestat, inefficient metabolism, the desire to celebrate good times, or the need to find solace in bad times, all boiled down to one basic but surprisingly often overlooked psychological principle. *And it is this principle that the Eating Man's Diet reverses and uses to your full advantage.*

Obviously there is no automatic "cure-all" in weight reduction programs, no matter how exciting a new concept may at first appear. (See Chapter Two: *The Gimmick Diets: Why They Work—Why They Don't,* and Chapter Three: *The No-Gimmick Diets: Why They Work—Why They Don't.*) Any weight loss requires effort, and any lasting loss requires *time* as well. The Eating Man's Diet, however, requires one thing more: *a full understanding of what makes it work and why it must work for you.*

Accordingly I've divided this book into short, easy-to-read chapters, intended to lead you in easy transitions from one concept to another, explaining the diet in detail and how, once its significant elements are grasped, you can then set up *your own customized version*. (With no two eating problems identical, does it make sense to construct identical weight reduction programs?) In the back you'll find an appendix containing suggested daily menus—which you are free to adapt to your own specifications—a weight chart, a calorie counter, and—very important—a listing of the approximate number of calories necessary to maintain you at your ideal weight.

Read the Eating Man's Diet carefully. Question its concepts as you go. Take none of them for granted. Remember: a complete absorption of its principles coupled with a real desire to reduce will not only help you to reach your ideal weight, it will provide you with the necessary insight into the *real* problems of weight reduction so that you may maintain that ideal weight—without hunger—for what in all probability will be a *happier, healthier and longer life.*

Good luck.

And good eating to you!

1

Is the "Eating Man's Diet" for You?

Not necessarily.

No diet is for you—without the approval of your physician. It happens that the "Eating Man's Diet" is one of the safest ever conceived. (An eminent professor at a British school of medicine has written: "As regards its safety, it should certainly be more desirable from this point of view than almost any other form of regimen yet proposed.") If you're a normally healthy person—aside from your weight problem—you should be able to undertake it without hazard. But let your physician decide.

No diet is for you—if you're simply looking for a free and easy ride. The "Eating Man's Diet" *is not easy*—because there is no easy diet. It will make considerable demands upon you. It will deprive you of food when you want it— and force food upon you when you'd just as soon pass it up. It will ask you to change habits, both of under- and overeating, that you have perhaps built up over a lifetime. True, it *does* seem to get easier as you go along. But the first three weeks are crucial. Our experience shows that *each person* who has stuck it out those first three weeks has continued to a significant and seemingly lasting weight loss. Some have insisted it's the easiest diet they've ever heard of. *Easiest* it may be . . . but that doesn't make it *easy*.

No diet is for you—if your entire objective is to "lose 10 pounds by next Tuesday." True, you can record a good-sized reduction in a short period of time (five to 10 pounds in one week is not uncommon). But you must realize that any such initial loss is largely of fluid. If it goes quickly, it can return just as quickly. *Any lasting weight loss takes time.*

Now, the "Eating Man's Diet" *is* for you—if you've always dreamed of becoming one of those marvelous people who seem to be able to eat anything they please while never gaining a pound.

The "Eating Man's Diet" *is* for you—if you rather like the idea of going out on dates, attending family parties, joining the girls (or boys) for a generous luncheon, or simply sitting down with your mate to a quiet supper *without passing up a single course from appetizer to dessert and in no way forming a guilty conscience because you've broken or cheated on your diet.*

The "Eating Man's Diet" *is* for you—if you've tried every other weight reduction program there is, both the so-called "gimmick" and "no-gimmick" diets, and found that however great they worked on paper, they simply didn't work on *you.*

The "Eating Man's Diet" *is* for you—if you've never tried another diet before.

Finally, the "Eating Man's Diet" *is* for you—if you are willing, on completing this book, to put aside whatever arguments you may be able to muster against it—however logical they might seem—and *invest the necessary three weeks* to begin your new lifelong eating habits. Although case after case bears us up, we cannot "prove" this revolutionary approach will work with *you.* This is something you will have to prove to *yourself.* And you can't prove—or disprove—it by thinking about it.

You'll have to try it.

For three weeks.

Give it that long—and *you'll know it works.* What's more, you will then be fully able to continue with it until your ideal weight is reached, knowing that once you get there you'll have so programmed your habits of eating that *you'll stay there.*

2

2

The "Gimmick" Diets: Why They Work— Why They Don't

Gimmick diets *do* work, you know.

They work superbly—for a short period of time. Then they stop working altogether.

What do we mean by gimmick diets? Basically, they might be defined as methods of weight reduction in which one particular type of food is emphasized (often in almost limitless quantities) above and beyond all others.

Thus we have the bananas and skimmed milk diet.

We have the cottage cheese diet.

We have the champagne (!) diet.

We have the all-protein . . . all-carbohydrate . . . and all-fat diet.

We have the rice diet . . . the liquid diet . . . and, in a slight departure from the above definition, we have the "countless calories" diet.

And they work! Every one of them.

But they *do* work only for a little while. They *can* be highly dangerous. And when they're completed, the weight that is lost is usually, and quickly, gained right back.

Before we examine why they *don't* work then, let's examine why they *do*.

The primary fact to remember in weight reduction (but a fact that is all too frequently forgotten) is that *any* decrease in daily calorie consumption is bound to bring about a weight loss—however temporary or fleeting.

Now one of the seemingly easiest ways to bring about a calorie decrease—which then forces the body to turn upon its fat deposits in order to fulfill its energy needs—is to emphasize one food above all others.

Why is this?

Because the body is able to tolerate only so much of a good (or bad) thing.

As an example, a "perfect" diet to a small child might be a limitless amount of sweets. (Or so the child may think.) Take a little boy to a baseball game or a circus. He'll want to order every time he sees the ice cream man, the cotton candy man, the caramel corn man and the soft drink man. Because it is, after all, a special occasion, an indulgent parent might cater to the child's whims too often. And what happens? The child is suddenly, gravely ill. He wants no part of sweets—or any other kind of food. And his system may well purge itself, most spectacularly, of those sweets he has already consumed.

Too much of a good thing.

An adult, on the other hand, is more capable of discerning how much his system is able to tolerate. Put an adult on nothing but bananas and skimmed milk and he soon hates the sight of both. Since the diet gives him no other choice of food, however, there is nothing for him to do but consume fewer calories than he otherwise would (assuming, of course, that he remains on this regimen). Thus he drops weight—often quite a bit.

A short time ago, a widely best-selling book (which was soon to be discredited) was based on the premise that one need not cut down on his calories at all—he had only to eat a good deal of polyunsaturated fat to become thin. Or so most people who had only casually read the book understood it. However, those who attempted the prescribed method soon became aware that they not only had to eat a good deal of polyunsaturated fat (actually recommended *to the point of nausea*), they also had to *cut down drastically* on their carbohydrate intake. (Among the counsels given was to never eat a piece of candy again—nor cake, nor ice cream, nor fruit juices, nor cookies, nor pastries, nor any kind of cream, nor sugar, nor sugar derivative, nor anything containing starch! And these were all to be eliminated not for their calorie content, you understand, but *because they contained carbohydrates*.) Did the diet work? You bet it did. And it worked for the same reason the other gimmick diets do . . . because it emphasized a particular food—literally, in this case—*ad nauseam.*

Now that we've seen why the gimmick diets *do* work, let's see why they *don't.*

First of all, most of them are based on the *crash* principle.

No sane man or woman is going to drink champagne—to the exclusion of all other liquids and foods—forever. For one thing, it's a bit expensive. More importantly, however, by eliminating the proteins, the vitamins, the carbohydrates and/or the fats the body daily requires to do its proper job, one places himself in grave danger of becoming seriously ill if the diet should continue for any length of time.

Therefore, one undertakes such a diet for only a short period. It's dandy if you're a jockey or a boxer and have to make a certain weight for a race or a fight. But—as jockeys and boxers know—once the event is over, the weight comes zooming back on.

Secondly, even if not based on a *crash,* such a diet bears so little similarity to what might be called "normal" eating that when one completes it and faces the world of *real food* once more, he has a sensation quite like that of an alcoholic who'd spent several weeks or months "drying out" and then was turned loose in a tavern with orders to "drink moderately." One drink—or one bite of food—leads to another and another and another. (The alcoholic, by the way, however much more painful his habit, does have at least one advantage over the dieter. At such a critical point he *does* have the option of refusing that first drink. The dieter, poor wretch, *must* begin eating again.)

Thus we see that the *non-crash* gimmick diet (as administered in institutions—supplemented, of course, by vitamin injections or their equivalent) often does no more lasting good than the *crash* gimmick diets. This is also true, of course, of the institutionalized "starvation" type of diet—which, supplemented by vitamin shots, has gotten a good deal of publicity in the last few years—and what is perhaps the most bizarre method of weight reduction of all: that of sewing the stomach closed so that all food, unaffected by digestive juices, travels directly into the small intestine, making calorie build-up a physical impossibility.

(The daughter of a noted Hollywood actor had such an operation—after years of extreme obesity. In a period of months the young woman lost all of her extra fat and achieved quite a flattering figure. At this point—so that she wouldn't starve—the doctors re-opened her stomach once more. She, of course, gained back every pound she'd lost.)

It might be a good idea to ponder, before moving on, why the men who conduct these diets—some of them quite brilliant and dedicated to their tasks—continue to prescribe such methods in the face of what obesity expert Dr. Stanley Schacter of Columbia University calls "the notorious long-run ineffectiveness of virtually all attempts to treat obesity."

One reason, of course, is that on occasion (as little as two per cent of the time, according to one estimate) the results in a particular case *do* prove lasting.*

Another is that the argument can be made that it is better to reduce a badly overweight person *even for a very short period* than never to reduce him at all. (This argument, of course, is subject to challenge.)

But the greatest *plus* in favor of their work—aside from, perhaps, the research value—would seem to be based on the commonly observed phenomenon that seriously overweight people are, in this respect at least, among the most hopeless individuals known. Like alcoholics, dope addicts or compulsive gamblers, they've a monkey on their back (nearly a literal thing here) which *they* don't fully understand—and which their friends, relatives, business associates and even personal physicians often can't begin to fathom. They come

---

* I commend to you a study by Haslim and Van Itallie of the Nutrition Clinic, St. Luke's Hospital, New York City, in which several obese patients were hospitalized and subjected—some for several months—to a diet of unlimited amounts of nutritious low-calorie liquid. The patients, having no choice but to drink this bland food or go without, lost impressive amounts of weight while in the hospital. Following their release, however, they regained *without exception* every single pound. (Annals of N. Y. Academy of Sciences 131, 654, 1965)

from all walks of life. They can be poor or rich, male or female, young or old, sick or (otherwise) healthy, intelligent or ignorant—a bustling, successful leader or a withdrawn, timid loser.

The doctors—and the victims—feel that if they can achieve a normal figure *once* . . . if one time in their lives they can look in the mirror without disgust, experience the sensory and mental pleasure of slipping into a trim, stylish fashion rather than the awkward embarrassment of tugging on a gunny sack with sleeves, discover the delight of bending without wheezing—or of charging up a flight of stairs without their hearts threatening to explode . . . they just *might* be so inspired as to somehow take whatever steps are necessary to maintain their newly found status quo.

And of course they try.

The doctors help them to try.

There are medicines prescribed and nutrients provided and excruciatingly detailed long-range eating plans devised.

But in the great majority of cases it is all to no avail.

What was lost in the institution is regained in the world outside—and all because of *one small but all-powerful factor that neither the doctors nor the patients seem to take into account* . . .

3

The "No-Gimmick" Diets: Why They Work —Why They Don't

No-gimmick diets also work, of course.

Given a choice between the two, the no-gimmick diets are usually held as greatly superior to the gimmick variety.

They don't seem to be intrinsically dangerous, for one thing—since they emphasize meals that are balanced in every respect but calories.

And it makes sense, after all, that by reducing calories one more-or-less automatically reduces his weight.*

Most doctors recommend them.

Most overweight people have tried them.

Indeed there is some evidence that scarcely a day goes by in the life of an obese person (or a thin one, for that matter) when he doesn't in some respect employ the precepts of the no-gimmicks. Anyone who has ever drunk his coffee black while preferring cream and sugar, ordered skimmed milk instead of whole, tossed off a diet cola instead of the regular, passed up ice cream in favor of an apple, or devoured a zesty, tangy, nutrition-packed salad while secretly craving a hot pastrami sandwich was—in a way—practicing those very precepts.

No-gimmick diets make so very much sense in fact, it's a wonder sometimes that there are any overweight people left.

* Incidentally, the word "calorie" need never be mentioned in these diets, some preferring to merely list "recommended" and "non-recommended" foods. But with the former relatively low in calories and the latter relatively high, they remain nonetheless low-calorie approaches.

Indeed, with all those who have tried them, there might *not* be—if they really worked.

But, like the gimmick variety, they really don't.

And contrary to what you may personally believe—especially if you've tried no-gimmick diets without success—*the failure is not in you at all . . . but in the diets themselves.*

As before, however, let's reserve our investigation into why they *don't* work until we see why they *do.*

No-gimmick diets *do* work because they are mathematically designed to allow you—on a regular basis—somewhat fewer calories than your body normally "burns."

On a typical "short term" program—one week, say—you'd be allowed as many as 900 calories a day. If your ordinary requirement was, for example, 2300 calories, you would show a net daily deficit of 1400, thereby losing nearly three pounds by the end of that week.

(The scale would probably show a greater loss but, as stated before, most of it would be fluid—and gained back very quickly. We'll examine the problem of how to tell the false loss—*or gain*—from the real in a later chapter.)

If you desired to lose more than three pounds, you would be well-advised to *increase* your daily consumption to 1200 calories. You could thus remain on the diet for two weeks—since it is generally not considered desirable to remain on a 900-calorie diet that long. Your second week, according to mathematics, would see you lose between two and two-and-a-half pounds.

Beyond two weeks a minimum of 1500 calories would be called for—unless, of course, you were under regular doctor's care and had an *urgent* reason for reducing more quickly. At 1500 calories daily you would lose about a pound-and-a-half a week. Truly, it doesn't sound like much, but it *does* represent 78 pounds in a year—were you to remain faithful to the diet that long.

And, of course, since this is a no-gimmick approach, you would be assured that what are usually considered your main nutritional needs—those of vitamins, proteins, iron, etc.—would be filled regularly. The no-gimmicks staunchly recommend foods such as beefsteak, chicken, seafoods and vegetables—which are chockful of these necessities—while

9

forbidding or severely restricting those rich in starch, sugar and fat—all of which are, of course, high in calories.

Now we can divide the no-gimmicks, for the sake of convenience, into three basic categories: One, the most common, is undertaken solely on your own (with, it is hoped, a doctor's formal or tacit approval); the second is with your physician's direct collaboration and supervision; the third— an increasingly popular way to attempt weight reduction— would find you dieting in concert with a group of heavy-weights.

Although there are no precise statistics to substantiate the comparative effectiveness of these methods, the second is generally thought to be much more successful than the first, and the third (often attempted by people who have tried— and failed at—the first and second) would seem to be about on par with, or somewhat more effective than, the second.

We've already seen why the simplest of the no-gimmicks (dieting on one's own) works. The second works for the same reason—i.e., the fact that it is mathematically and nutritionally correct. It has, however, a wealth of additional factors going for it:

Dieting with a doctor works because of the regularity— whether weekly or monthly—of the visits that *must be made*. (You've contracted, at least psychologically, to see him at an appointed time regardless of reduction or gain. With the commitment made, you feel you'd *better* show a reduction.)

Dieting with a doctor works because of his professional ability to inspire confidence in the program you are under-taking (and, often, his ability to put the fear of God into you if you are slipshod in your performance).

Dieting with a doctor works because *it costs you money*. No one likes to throw money away—and that's just what you do if you can't somehow attain good results. It is for this reason that, often, the more it costs—the better your results are.

Dieting with a doctor works because he can—and often does—prescribe pills to help you along in your program. These may encompass anything from vitamins and diuretics to appetite depressants and tranquilizers. (Unfortunately, some so-called "diet doctors" have been known to prescribe these—and more questionable medications—excessively and indiscriminately. But such conduct, however reprehensible, would seem to be the exception rather than the rule. Under the direction of a competent physician, the pills *can* be an aid to maintaining a weight reduction program.)

Finally, dieting with a doctor works because of the nature of the dieter himself. The majority of overweight people never bother—because of the expense, the embarrassment, or their own plain lethargy—to seek the direct guidance of a physician. The minority who do therefore demonstrate both a greater concern and a certain resolve or determination to Do Something about their condition. Such resolve, however unsteady, is the necessary big first step in any program.

This brings us to the group diets.

Based on some of the same principles that have proven "the last best hope" in such organizations as Alcoholics Anonymous and, lately, Synanon, the group diets work for many of the same reasons the physician-supervised diets do —that is, the regularity of the meetings, the confidence inspired (and fear of failure engendered) by the chapter's director and/or one's fellow dieters, the fact of money outlay, and the particular nature of the minority of overweight people who subscribe to these groups: they're often *more* concerned—and therefore determined—than those entering the doctor's office.

However, the basic—and differentiating—factor in this approach's favor is the twofold essence of group psychology:

On the one hand you have "receiving-end" help. That is, when you're down and out, you've a buddy to help pick you up; when you feel it absolutely can't be done, there are a dozen people to tell you that they, indeed, have done it; when you're ready to chuck the whole thing, almost any member can tell you he once felt exactly the same way— *but he stuck it out.*

On the other hand—and more importantly—the group diets, unlike any other type already mentioned, provide help by putting you on the "giving end" as well. That is, as you find yourself conforming to your chapter's standards, as you begin to realize some weight loss and satisfaction in your progress, you are encouraged—and in fact feel the need—to pass some of the lessons you have learned along to some of the newer and more unfortunate members. However un-

11

selfish may be your motives, you actually derive more benefit from this good counsel than those you are attempting to help. For as we teach, so do we learn. No argument makes so much sense as does the argument from your own lips. Intellectually persuaded at the start, you are emotionally convinced when you are through.

The group diet—when you're ready for it—is indeed "the last best hope," preferable, in this writer's opinion, to any we've so far discussed.

But, as I said before, it really doesn't work.

None of the no-gimmick approaches work on the majority of fat people. If they did, there just wouldn't be so many fat people around (and statistics show that their percentage of the population is increasing, not declining).

Of course, it can be argued that, as Chesterton once observed about the Christian ideal, the diets haven't failed— it's just that they've been "left untried."

Such an argument, however, is simply not consistent with statistics or common observation.

Americans—and others fortunate enough to live in prospering countries—are attempting to diet today in numbers unprecedented in the history of man. Until only very recently the situation was exactly reversed. People were (and, sadly, now *are*—in many parts of the world) trying to *gain* weight, to find *enough* to eat, not concerned with what to do with an *excess* of nutriment.

The financial page of your newspaper will show that new low-calorie foods—from complete, canned meals and liquid lunches to sugarless gum and carbohydrate-free beer—are being taken off the grocery shelves as rapidly as they're introduced. Indeed, special sections devoted to diet foods have become standard in the supermarkets in only the last three years. One artificial sweetener manufacturer proudly claims his product, in one form or another, can be found in virtually every American kitchen. And the *accessories* to weight reduction sell as never before. They range from stationary (and mobile) bicycles to sweatsuits, electric vibrators and built-in sauna baths.

As clothing manufacturers cut waistbands and collars larger and larger, as airlines, movie houses and ball parks replace narrow seats with steadily wider ones, as heart doctors thunder against the danger of excessive weight and presidents establish councils on physical fitness—Americans diet . . . and diet . . . and diet.

But the sad fact is: Few of them ever succeed at reaching their ideal weight level. And of the handful who do, not a thimbleful manage to stay there.

We saw in the previous chapter that most gimmick diets fail because their basic plans are so far removed from ordinary, everyday eating.

It shouldn't be too surprising therefore to learn that *the no-gimmicks fail for exactly the same reason.*

It's true. As close to "normal" diets as they seem—full of vitamins, proteins, minerals, carbohydrates and even fats —balanced in all respects but calories—that single omission, the lack of sufficient units of energy to sustain one's normal weight level, renders them quite as ineffective as the gimmicks.

Anyone who ever embarks on a weight reduction program necessarily does so not with one—but with two distinct goals in mind.

How are you ever going to lose weight and maintain your loss if the diets—gimmick and no-gimmick—*absolutely refuse to take one of these goals into consideration?*

4

The Twin Goals of Weight Reduction: Why Reducing Is Never Enough

When you embark on a diet, you do so with *two* objectives in mind—whether you realize it or not.

The first, obviously, is to take off some weight: to remove excess fat in a safe and sane manner. You'll want to do this as quickly as possible without jeopardizing your health, alienating your family and friends through irritability, or causing your skin to sag by losing the fat beneath it faster than its natural elasticity can cope with. Hand in hand with the idea of *taking* it off goes the idea of *keeping* it off when the diet is ended.

The second objective, quite distinct but equally important, is to somehow find *freedom from hunger* along the way.

When you think in terms of a *new you,* after all, the picture you have in mind is of more than just a slimmer person wearing nicer clothes and looking more attractive. You also must see yourself as *enjoying* all this. And you know you can't enjoy it if you're continually hungry.

A *new you,* to be a viable conception, must feel at ease on your new daily eating regimen. If you are to consume no more than, say, 2300 calories daily for the rest of your life, *you will have to accept this fact both mentally and emotionally.*

Consuming 2300 calories per day really isn't so bad, after

14

all. There are millions of people in this country who willingly consume no more than that. They "burn" 2300 calories daily, so they eat 2300 calories daily. They don't gain or lose weight. And they're not hungry.

And they're not fat.

"Ah! To be one of those lucky millions!," you may think. "I'd be thin today myself except that—"

Here the excuses differ.

One may say (as I've said): "I was born heavy. My mother constantly overfed me. I continued to eat too much as an adult and I've now developed a dependence on food which would make life pretty bleak if I were to cut down on it."

Another may say: "I was a great athlete as a young man (or young woman). I was always burning excessive amounts of energy, so naturally I had to eat excessive amounts of food. As I grew older, however, I cut down on my physical activity without appreciably reducing my food intake. I just wouldn't know what to do if I had to try to get by with less than I'm eating now."

A third excuse involves the "appestat"—that is, the control center in your brain that tells you when you've had "enough." The excuse runs: "My appestat just doesn't function properly. It never says *enough* until I know I've had *too much*. When I try to eat what everybody else does and no more—I just go hungry."

Yet another excuse is concerned with basal metabolism—the basic rate at which your body burns energy aside from any physical activity on your part. "My rate is low," one person may say. "It really isn't that I eat so very much. What I *do* eat is converted into fat instead of being used up."

This last excuse is about on par with those of "glands" and "heredity." Scientifically discredited time and again, it remains popular with a certain number of would-be weight watchers simply because there *is* some truth that any of these three *can* be a factor in obesity. However, they apply to only a small percentage of those who are overweight. Furthermore, it's been shown that proper diet will aid in reducing *anybody*—none of these excuses withstanding.

There are, after all, a great number of people with low basal metabolism, a heritage of obesity or even defective glands *who are not fat.* The proper treatment for any true physical disorder, however, is in the doctor's office and is beyond the scope of this book.

Whatever your excuse may be, however, for "needing" excessive amounts of food on a daily basis, modern psychology realizes the immediate, causative reason for your eating too much is the same, exact reason you have for scratching your nose (if you do), or cracking your knuckles, or putting on your left shoe before your right shoe, or tugging at an ear lobe or rising on a certain side of the bed.

You perform any one of these physical mannerisms or traits *today* because you did so *yesterday*—and the day before, and the day before.

Dr. Freud notwithstanding, a host of modern psychologists and psychiatrists seek not so much to treat the *origin* of the act as much as they do its *habituation.*

Your slim neighbor down the street may have problems almost identical to yours. At times he may be nervous, irritable, fearful or depressed—but he does not overeat in order to live with these problems.

Of course not. Why should he?

He *didn't* overeat yesterday—or the day before, or the day before. Taking in excessive food as a solution just never even occurs to him.

Ask yourself this question in all seriousness: *If* you were thin—right now, and *if* you had been thin for the past couple of years, and *if* over all this time you had eaten no more than your allotted 2300 or 2700 or 3400 calories per day through all the highs and lows I'm sure you've experienced, *do you honestly believe* that if a crisis situation were to arise at this minute you would attempt to solve it by *overeating?*

In all probability your answer will be no. And even if it *isn't*—if you're so accustomed to overeating in a crisis situation that you honestly feel you just might go on a binge under the circumstances described above—in all probability you wouldn't anyhow. Having formed sound habits of regular, normal eating over an extended period of time, there's little if any doubt that you would continue to stick with these habits, reacting to crisis or severe temptation almost identically like those who had never had a weight problem.

For that is the only basic difference between you and the "normal." They've habituated themselves to sound eating; you've habituated yourself to excessive eating.

They have found *freedom from hunger*—which is not to say that they don't at times find themselves severely hungry and tempted to eat too much. They do—but their habit helps them to control such urges.

Your *freedom from hunger,* on the other hand, still waits in the undetermined future.

Make no mistake about it. *Freedom from hunger* is quite as important an objective in a sound diet program as is the actual reduction itself. Hunger, as defined by Webster's Third International Dictionary, is "a craving, desire, *or* urgent need for food." (My emphasis.) This craving, this desire or this urgent need—whether physical, emotional, or a combination of the two—is what started your weight problem in the first place.

If it *weren't* for hunger, you could have adopted any sound low calorie plan long ago and carried it off successfully.

If not for hunger, there'd be no doubt that when you completed such a plan you would remain at your ideal weight without difficulty.

However, as you well know, hunger is not so easily banished.

And no one would expect it to be.

This signal within us, this crying out for food, is as vital an impulse as that which cries out for breath.

Schacter calls it *"the most primitive of motives."*

Joseph Conrad, an author celebrated for his deep psychological insights into man, said the following about hunger's driving, compelling force:*

"No fear can stand up to hunger, no patience can wear it out, disgust simply does not exist where hunger is; and as to superstition, beliefs, and what you may call principles, they are less than chaff in a breeze."

Try pitting hunger against the actuarial tables of your insurance company, which say that your life expectancy is

---

* *Heart of Darkness,* used with permission of J. M. Dent & Sons, Ltd., London, England, and the Trustees of the Joseph Conrad Estate.

greatly shortened if you remain overweight. Who wins? *"No fear can stand up to hunger . . ."*

Climb aboard a crash diet. Undereat day after day after day. Hang in there. This time you won't give in. You're going to battle hunger and *win,* you tell yourself, if you can just hold on long enough. *"No patience can wear it out . . ."*

How could I have eaten that much last night? *How could I?,* you wonder. Well, that's the last time. I'll never gorge like that again. I'm so disgusted—! *"Disgust simply does not exist where hunger is . . ."*

Well, I don't care. I've made up my mind this time. I'm going to stick with my diet, no matter what. I've told all my friends. I've warned my family. I've practically taken a vow. *". . . and as to superstition, beliefs, and what you may call principles, they are less than chaff in a breeze."*

This is the enemy, the enemy each of us must fight: hunger.

And it is by no means an easy enemy.

But you've got to beat it if you're going to reduce and stay reduced.

The only real way to do that, however, is to *satisfy* it.

5

You Are Not a "Foodaholic" and Should Never Be Treated Like One

"Satisfy hunger?," you may ask. "Isn't this, in a sense, like giving in? After all, other 'addictions'—drugs, for instance, or alcohol, or tobacco—are often best treated by *never* satisfying them. Can't we apply somewhat the same principles here?"

Unfortunately, no. We can't.

There's been a good deal written lately comparing the addictions mentioned here to the habit of overeating. (I myself, to make a point, offered a comparison between the *victims* in Chapter Two.) But whatever the similarities between the obese and, say, the alcoholic, their *problems* remain entirely different.

Alcoholism is, in all respects, an *addiction*.

Consistent overeating, however, is not. As severe as it may be, it remains nothing but a *bad habit*.

Now what is the basic difference between the two? Are we merely, after all, playing with words?

NO. THE TWO ARE ENTIRELY DISSIMILAR. AND THEY NEVER VARY SO MUCH AS THEY DO IN THEIR TREATMENT.

A great deal that is wrong with most attempts to treat obesity lies in the confusion between this problem and addiction. A pair of illustrations, however, will show you just how vast the gap between them is.

Joe K. is a heavy smoker who finally decided to overcome

19

his problem. He made up his mind to elminate tobacco from his life.

Now his first day was very rough indeed. He had grave doubts that he would ever get through it. But somehow he succeeded.

The next couple of days were also very rough—almost as bad as the first. But he'd been told that the initial three-day period was the hardest of all. With great difficulty he managed to continue to abstain during the entire period, looking forward to the fourth day as being somehow *easier*.

And it was. Not as easy as he'd hoped—but easier.

So it went for six weeks or so, easier day following easier day.

When six weeks had elapsed, give or take a couple of days, Joe knew he had the problem licked.

The addiction was gone.

The habit was gone. (All addictions can be categorized as habit; the reverse, however, does not follow.)

Joe knew it remained possible for him to begin smoking again—but to do so he would have to form a *new* addiction or habit. He had licked the addiction he'd had.

Mary B., on the other hand, is obese—a heavy eater.

One day she also decided to overcome her problem. She laid out a diet plan for herself and made up her mind that she would stick to it.

Now Mary's first day—unlike Joe's—was not really so bad. Indeed, she didn't expect it would be. She'd often managed to diet for a day or so in the past. Her crisis, she knew, was yet to come.

The second day was just a little harder than the first—and the third day was *very* hard. But Mary had, as we've noted, "made up her mind." She clung on, although the diet sometimes seemed to grow more trying by the hour.

In her case, six weeks also passed. And she persevered! But Mary well knew that as each day progressed into each succeeding day, the diet became more and more difficult.

When six weeks were gone, Mary was ready to go berserk —and she did, in a grand eating binge that she would long remember.

Unlike Joe, she had had to schedule a three-month period of deprivation (30 pounds were her goal, and she had planned to lose them at what is about the maximum rate: 2½ pounds per week). She'd lost only 15 of those pounds by the end of her sixth week.

By the end of her eighth week, all 15 were back with her again.

The basic difference between Joe's battle and Mary's should be very easy to spot.

When you eliminate an addiction—as stubborn as it may be—time becomes your ally. You reach a critical point early in your effort and then, with each passing day, your task becomes less and less difficult.

When you attempt to treat a weight problem in the same way, however, time becomes your enemy. The "critical point" lies far in the distant future—if indeed it's *ever* reached—and your task, as each day passes, becomes *harder*.

Fortunately for Joe, he could take on his crisis right at the beginning when his determination and resolve were at their peak. Once it had passed, he had only to live from one day to the next, allowing the formidable strength of habit to form.

Unfortunately for Mary, her determination and resolve were strongest when the problem was easiest. They declined as the problem increased—and somehow *habit never did seem to form!* (We'll see, as a matter of fact, that under the circumstances it was *psychologically impossible* for Mary to use habit as an aid in her quest.)

No, the methods of treating addiction are *not* the methods to treat obesity. "Foodaholic," in addition to being a clumsy word, is essentially meaningless. It is as impossible to "addict" yourself to food as it is to "addict" yourself to air and water.

Alcohol, tobacco, drugs—none of these are basic necessities to life.

Food, air and water are.

And there lies all the difference.

6

The Search for a Better Diet— a Physical Clue

Suppose for a minute that someone were to suddenly, forcefully attempt to cut off your air supply. Would you fight?

Suppose you were attending the Inaugural Ball at the time of the attack—or singing at Sunday services . . . Suppose you were only half awake just prior to it . . . Do you believe you'd allow any of these factors to prevent you from an immediate, all-out response?

Would it make any conceivable difference to you what goals, thoughts or plans you had had in mind immediately beforehand?

Of course not. You'd fight without hesitation, without embarrassment, without quarter—and *with or without conscious decision*—until at last your air supply was restored.

It's that important to you. Nothing else matters—or *can* matter. Even if you're a normally timid, forebearing person, your body is quite prepared to act "as if with a will of its own" to keep the passage between your lungs and the life-giving oxygen outside open and functioning.

Such are the instincts provided by the Creator in all air-breathing animals. Your body, needing air to continue living, does not have to wait for a command from your consciousness to begin the job of defending and preserving itself. Indeed it will vigorously oppose all conscious commands to the contrary. (It is for this reason that doctors are able to

22

readily dismiss the fears of parents whose children threaten to hold their breath until they "turn blue." Either the child will become so uncomfortable that he'll give up the game himself or, in a radical case, the body will allow a temporary *loss of consciousness* so that the *subconscious*—our automatic mechanisms—can take over and restore breathing.) When it comes to air, the body simply will not allow you to say *no*.

Not so surprisingly, quite the same principle applies to food.

Certainly you *can* cut down on food for a time (just as you are able to hold your breath). But your body reaches a certain point wherein its immediate supply—that is, the readily available blood sugar—nears exhaustion. At this point, if you are to continue to live, the body is forced to begin feeding upon itself. *And this is something your body objects violently to doing.*

We're taught in school that fat is "stored" in order to provide the body with an ever-ready source of energy. This is true as it stands. Your body, however, does not quite "see" it that way.

It would seem to be very much a *miser* with all it stores. Let it put away 15 pounds of fat or 150. When you seek to retrieve and use some of these deposits, the body becomes equally disagreeable in both cases. Indeed, it's easily seen that if the objection were not the same, it would be far easier for a man severely overweight to reduce than one who was only moderately fat. In a case where the difference was between 150 and 15 pounds of surplus, the grossly overweight man would not begin to experience the difficulties of the thinner man until he'd already dropped 135 pounds!

(I must parenthetically note here that such a severely overweight person can *seem* to lose 15 pounds or so with astonishing ease. But, as mentioned before, an "easy" loss—such as he might sustain during a session in a steam room—represents water, not fat, and is rapidly recovered. In the context of this book, losing "weight" means the removal of excess fat.)

However, anyone who is quite heavy knows that it does not make much difference how much your body has put away before you begin your diet. As soon as you start to withdraw these stores, your body begins its objections—by sending increasingly persistent "hunger signals" into your consciousness. Such signals may be the generally accepted "growling stomach" or a feeling of weakness caused by a reduction of sugar in the blood. Or, as investigators have found out, your feeling of hunger may not be physically evident at all—that is, the most sophisticated examinations often cannot find any association between what is known as "physiological hunger" and the perhaps vague feeling of discomfort—the "craving or desire" for food—that an extremely overweight person may justifiably—albeit subjectively—label as *hunger*.*

The point is, your body does not like to go without calories any more than it likes to go without air. It not only objects (through cries of hunger) as you force it to withdraw its stores, it would also seem to "keep records" as to exactly how much you have had it withdraw!

If you've been halfway successful with any diet in the past, you have experienced this "record-keeping."

Lose five pounds on a diet and when does your body stop crying hunger? When you've gained each of the five pounds back.

Lose 15 pounds—and does your body stop crying hunger when you regain five? You know it doesn't. You remain vaguely uncomfortable—your appetite aroused and constantly tempting you to overeat—until you've gained all 15 back (and perhaps a little more).

And so it goes if your loss is 30 pounds or whatever.

Again, to use the air analogy, what do you do if you've been holding your breath for any considerable length of time —say a minute or two—when at last you make oxygen available to yourself once again? Resume breathing "normally"? You do not. You pant, you gasp, you gulp the air down. Your body would seem to play along with you as you deprive it of oxygen for a time. As soon as the deprivation is ended, however, it insists that the "loss" is quickly made up.

* Albert Stunkard, M.D. of the University of Pennsylvania and Hilde Bruch, M.D. of Baylor University have done some impressive work along this line. (A. Stunkard, Psychosomatic Medicine, 21, 281, 1959: H. Bruch, Psychiatric Quarterly, 35, 458, 1961.)

I admit I've painted a pretty dreary picture of what may at first glance seem to be the body's "insane" desire to retain the *status quo* at all costs.

However, it can be seen that such a determined impulse could well have proven to be one of man's principal assets in the millions of years he has been upon this earth—only 5000 of which have been recorded or "civilized."

In the great bulk of his existence man has not had a readily available food supply. With no knowledge of farming or husbandry he has had to make a constant search for food. With no knowledge of food preservation, he could not lay aside what he found or killed. His only course was to use himself as a storehouse for it. In order to exist, his body would have had to prompt him to "overeat."

Too much overeating would have, of course, been a liability rather than an asset—perhaps even more so than it is today. In a climate or season where food was easy to come by, continual overeating would not be necessary.

How then would man's body (not, as we've seen, trusting to his intellect) tell him when he'd had enough?

Simple. It would base the amount needed to satisfy him upon *what had recently been his greatest weight.*

Thus when the hunter went out to hunt a deer, he might be forced to spend a week or two in extreme privation. Capturing his deer, he would proceed to make up for that week or two—and then, spurred by the "ghost appetite"— the sense of hunger that urges us to eat more even when it can be proven we have no physiological need for it *(at least right now),* he would proceed to eat somewhat in excess of his body's immediate physical demands, thereby insuring himself against starvation should his next deer take some-what longer to catch.

If he lost only a couple of pounds, say, while on the hunt, his body—not being greatly alarmed—would only urge him to put a couple back on.

If he lost 10, however, his body might urge he restore 12.

If he lost 15, his body might not declare itself "satisfied" until he had restored 20!

Pure speculation? Of course.

But we can see the pattern repeated even today in the case of hibernating animals.

A bear wakes up hungry from his long winter's nap. Does he find a quiet pool, admire his new-found slenderness and promise himself he'll remain at this weight? If he did, he wouldn't last through another winter. His life-preserving instinct prompts him to continually "overeat"—larding himself with pound upon pound of extra fat until such time as food is once more in short supply. Well-prepared, he can afford to "diet"—that is, let the body feed upon itself—until such time as food becomes plentiful again. And then, of course, his instinct prompts him to "overeat" once more.

Indeed, the story of the hunter—reflecting problems so deeply rooted and close to life's most basic instincts that science is thus far unable to offer physiological explanation for the undeniably existing "ghost appetite"*—would seem to explain two of the thorniest and most puzzling problems that continually plague the obese.

One is the well known Vicious Circle of under- and overeating the obese have long found themselves prey to. Just as the hunter, they may find themselves *undereating* for several days in a row. (It is during such a period they complain that they "don't eat any more than anybody else does." Indeed, if they were to conscientiously keep track of their calories during those days, they'd probably find they ate considerably *less*.) This period is, of course, followed by binge overeating. Having actually *lost some weight* (although their scales may not reflect the loss, their water being diverted to temporarily replace the few ounces or pounds that are missing), they proceed to make up for the loss—and gain a little more—until such time as they return to what they believe is "normal eating" again.

(To digress for just a moment, I've long been amazed at the considerable knowledge of nutrition and diet that most of the obese seem to have. The thought persists that if perhaps they had never originally *tried* to diet, if they *hadn't* been warned by a loving mother that a cherry cobbler contains four times the calories of a raw apple, if they *didn't* in fact attempt to cut calories whenever feasible—they might never have gotten into the *undereat* end of the cycle and therefore been spared the *overeat* end.)

* For an interesting discussion of some of the lengths the experts have gone to in studying this problem, see S. Schacter, Science, 161, 751, 1968.

The second puzzler our hypothetical hunter seems to solve is the apparent ease with which the obese are able to enter upon diets of pure starvation . . . and the fantastic difficulty they have of *not* overdoing it when the floodgates of food are wide open.

In my own case, when the potato chip commercial defied me that I "can't eat just one," I'd often—before discovering this diet—been forced to ruefully agree, knowing the struggle I had to eat "just one" of anything!

It's generally much easier for the obese to skip a meal entirely than it is for them to attempt to eat no more than normal portions.

And those who have been clinically "starved" report that it really isn't hard at all after the first few days.

Why is it we can do *without* but have such a hard time doing *with?*

Look at the hunter. What possible purpose would his hunger instinct achieve if it were to continue to progressively make his life miserable when food was just unavailable? He *knows* he's hungry. His body serves no useful function in constantly reminding him of it.

But—when he starts to eat! *Now* the appetite comes out. In order to make up for past hunger and ward off future, he is told to eat and eat and eat.

And, while we're at it, look at the bear. If his body were to barrage him with signals of hunger while he was hibernating, he'd get precious little sleep. His body would, in fact, be defeating its own purpose.

It waits until he awakens—and food is plentiful—before liberating his "bearlike" appetite!

I believe it can be seen from all the above that the problem of weight reduction—from a purely physical standpoint —is hardly well handled by the so-called "normal" or "logical" approaches to diet that we've previously discussed.

When you try to reduce you're doing battle with neither a calm intelligence nor a machine—either of which might possibly respond to the eminently "rational" approaches that have been foisted on us poor victims in the past, some of which I cite here:

"Eat less—weigh less."

"Cut calories—cut pounds."

"The world's best exercise is shaking your head from side

to side while slowly pushing away from the table when dessert is passed."

Such advice, however apparently sensible, has done little more for us than add guilt feelings to an already complex problem. Ignorant of the body's willful drive to keep firm hold on every pound it has, we've tried the "rational" approaches and failed miserably at them, being forced to con-
. clude in the face of such rationality that there must therefore be something *wrong with us*—physically, mentally, or morally (hence the myriad of oft refuted but persistent excuses).

We didn't know that we were only responding in the same manner anybody (or *any body*) would respond in similar circumstances.

We didn't realize that it is not a calm intelligence or machine we face but a totally unintelligent, quite irrational *subconscious drive toward life* which is so determined on protecting us it will kill us, if necessary, in order to do it.

And yet, even as the problem is defined, the answers begin to suggest themselves. The Vicious Circle of dieting . . . the fact that the very heavy have less difficulty in doing *without* than they have in doing *with** . . . the fact that dieting for a single day is not really that difficult, whereas dieting for an extended time *is* . . .

And perhaps most noteworthy of all: the fact that we are not simply dealing with the intellect here, nor even the body as such—but with a *subconscious drive* . . .

Add all these clues together and the answer is no longer so remote.

Of course, since it *is* the subconscious we are dealing with, it follows that the answer must not simply be a physical system but an intensely *psychological* one as well.

---

* In the introduction I postulated the idea that the overweight have a good deal more will power when it comes to abstaining from food than do the thin. The previously mentioned article by Schacter refers to a study conducted by himself and two colleagues—R. Goldman and M. Jaffa—which would seem to support this paradox. On Yom Kippur the orthodox Jew is supposed to fast for 24 hours. One's first inclination might be to think that the obese would prove much less successful at this attempt than the normal. Yet of the nearly 300 examined, only 68.8 per cent of the normal fasted—whereas 83.3 per cent of the obese made it through the full 24 hours!

7

The Search for
a Better Diet—
the Psychological Key

Of all the difficulties implicit in being overweight, none is harder to contend with than the enigma of habit.

It can be seen to be habit, after all (acting through hunger), that prompts those who are overweight to constantly repeat their eating patterns.

At the same time it's also habit that protects the normal from overeating in reaction to stress as do the obese.

It is habit that is the immediate, causative reason for *anyone's* daily living conventions—and more and more of today's psychologists are beginning to believe that *whatever its origins,* best results in treating an undesirable habit are usually obtained if it can be attacked *directly*—thus de-emphasizing the clinicians' familiar concern with problems of puberty or childhood that may have led to the habit's being formed.

The Duke of Wellington's famous remark—"Habit a second nature? Habit is ten times nature!"—remains the truest of truisms.

Yet it is habit that is ignored, overlooked and dismissed in virtually every diet plan!

Now it can be argued that other diets *do* attempt to deal with this phenomenon. They urge you, some of them, to "begin forming sound eating habits." Their first order of business, however, is to remove your excess weight.

Right. And this is precisely why they fail.

29

One half century ago William James, dean of American psychologists, dealt with the problem of habit in his book, *Psychology: Briefer Course,* in such a manner as to single out the reason for "the notorious long-range ineffectiveness of virtually all attempts to treat obesity"—if only nutritionists had had a mind to look for that reason at the time.

As Professor Willim S. Verplanck, head of the University of Tennessee's Department of Psychology, points out, it is possible to update James' words in the manner of the new technical terminology, but "the principle (like most of what William James wrote) is still good as gold."

Here's what James said:*

"In the main . . . all expert opinion would agree that abrupt acquisition of the new habit is the best way, *if there be a real possibility of carrying it out.* We must be careful not to give the will so stiff a task as to insure its defeat at the outset; but *provided one can stand it,* a sharp period of suffering and then a free time is the best thing to aim at, whether in giving up a habit like that of opium, or in simply changing one's hours of rising or of work."

Now I happened to be musing over that quote one day when the startlingly simple reason occurred to me why I— and the great majority of the overweight—failed at weight reduction programs time and again despite our best intentions and efforts.

It was because the diets we tried were not only *not* based on habit—*they were, in fact, so designed as to preclude the possibility of habit being formed!*

The idea may at first sound fantastic, but let's check the typical low calorie approach against James' criteria.

Using myself as an example, I am now at (or perhaps just slightly below) my "ideal weight." Standing 5'10" with unusually large bone structure—as demonstrated by my hat size of 7¾ and shoe size of 12EEE—I weigh in at 160 pounds.

In order to maintain my weight at 160, it is necessary for me to consume somewhere between 2400 and 3200 calories

---

* Used with permission of Holt, Rinehart & Winston, Inc., New York, N. Y.

30

daily.* Yet—back when I weighed 230—the *typical diet* would have immediately plunged me onto a daily consumption of 900 to 1500 calories, less than half of what I would *normally* require.

Of course it's clear enough that medication, hospitalization, group goals or sheer perseverance *might* have made it possible for me to consume so few calories over an extended period of time.

Yet no real habit would be formed.

I simply cannot exist indefinitely on less than half the calories I should be consuming . . .

There is therefore *no real possibility of carrying it out!*

Without that possibility, as James points out, there is *no possibility of habit* either.

On completion of such a program (whether prematurely or not) I would have developed no *new* habit—and therefore would still be saddled with my *old* habit: that of overeating.

That habit, coupled with the "ghost appetite" to be found at the terminus of such diets, would soon boost me up to 230 again.

James' keen insight into the problem of habit in turn gave *me* the insight that if I were ever to lick the problem of obesity it would have to be by throwing all the "rules" away and starting from the very beginning *with a diet firmly rooted on the habit principle.*

---

* The rule of thumb to determine your maintenance number of calories is to multiply the weight you seek to maintain by 15 or 20, depending on your physical activity. A more exact determination will be found in the appendix of this book.

8

The Secret—At Last

The first thing that occurred to me, as I sought to blend weight reduction with formation of lasting habit, was to select the number of calories needed to sustain me at my ideal weight and then simply consume that number on a regular day-in, day-out basis. In other words, since I then considered the "ideal" to be about 169 pounds,* I could therefore consume up to 3400 calories each day, form good habits and lose a little weight at the same time.

This "solution" had two distinct drawbacks, however.

One, obviously, was that losing weight in such a manner would take a long, long time.

The second was the very real possibility that I might not lose any weight at all! The rule of thumb of multiplying the weight you seek to maintain by 15 or 20 daily calories is precisely—and only—that: a rule of thumb. Suppose I were not as active as I imagined and I should have emphasized the 15 figure instead of the 20? Not even the Food and Nutrition Board of the National Academy of Sciences—who have prepared tables on the ideal number of calories to be

---

* The 169 figure may indeed be the "ideal," by the way. I only decided to lose the nine additional pounds after the diet had formally ended. I did this 1) to prove to myself that I was completely untroubled by "ghost appetite" (they came off quite easily); and 2) to provide a little buffer zone—*just in case.*

allowed for various weights and ages—can do any better than *estimate* the number of calories an individual should consume. With the diet to continue seemingly indefinitely, it might be several weeks—or months—before I discovered my mistake.

No, to be practicable, the diet would not only have to be habit-forming but relatively fast.

And suddenly I had the answer!

Have you ever *jogged?*

I don't mean run, trotted, or walked very quickly. I mean *jogged.*

Assuming for the moment that you haven't, let me tell you a little about *jogging's* principles:

Unlike any other form of popular exercise, jogging is based squarely on a 50-50 proposition.

Joggers work out one day and rest the next.

Even during the actual exercise 50-50 is the rule. The great majority of us are too far out of shape to simply run a couple of miles. And walking a couple, while good in itself, is not nearly as beneficial. Therefore, a jogger will *run* so many paces, *walk* so many paces, *run* so many paces, *walk* so many paces—*and find he can continue along this plan about as long as he wishes.*

There is no pain associated with jogging—and no strain either. It's strongly recommended for young and old alike (with, of course, their physician's approval)—*even,* and perhaps *especially,* for those with a history of heart trouble!

Besides all this, it is generally recognized as the *fastest* way to travel on foot between any two distant points. (You try to walk the distance and it'll take you forever; try running it and you'll soon fall over, exhausted.)

Jogging—or as I'd first heard it called as a youth: "boy-scout pacing"—was founded on sure physiological and psychological principles. In the brief time since it was first widely popularized through the book by William J. Bowerman and W. E. Harris, M.D.,* literally hundreds of thousands of people—some of whom had practically given up

---

* *Jogging,* published by Grosset & Dunlap, Inc., New York, N. Y., in association with *This Week Magazine.*

on any further attempt at physical conditioning—have bene-
fited dramatically from those principles.

What, I thought, *if I were to apply the very same principles to dieting?*

Of course! It was *the* answer.

The long-long-term program of consuming a regular 3400
calories per day was obviously unworkable. It would take
forever—like walking. And yet any attempt I'd ever made
(and I'd made quite a few) to consume a severely restricted
number of calories soon caused me to "fall over, exhausted"
—like running.

But to combine the two on a regular, every-other-day
basis!

Why, wasn't this exactly what James had suggested: "A
sharp period of suffering and then a free time"?!

"Abrupt acquisition of the new habit" just did not work
in the case of diet. As James said, it could only work "if
there be a real possibility of carrying it out." It was entirely
"so stiff a task as to insure its defeat at the outset."

But the body—as James and jogging's advocates long
realized—could readily, easily and even *habitually* function
on the premise of "a sharp period of suffering and then a
free time."

The concept was far different—both physically and psychologically—from trying to trot or diet indefinitely at, say,
three-quarters' speed . . . despite the fact that a full trot
combined with a walk—or a stiff diet combined with an
easy maintenance one—would seem to "logically" add up to
the same thing. (Later we'll review a couple of expert
opinions as to *why* this great difference should exist.)

And certainly the "day-on, day-off" principle would seem
to answer such problems we've discussed as *the Vicious
Circle of dieting* (basically by "harnessing," if you will, this
common trait among the obese: letting them still eat big and
eat small, but in such a manner as to *lose* rather than *gain*
weight), the fact that it's often easier to do *without* than
with (by allowing them to do *without* for a specific time and
then forcing them to do *with*—a most important consideration as Verplanck points out in Chapter 10), and finally
the fact that almost *no* obese person has real difficulty in
dieting for a single day ("Anyone," said Robert Louis

Stevenson, "can carry his burden, however hard, until night-fall. Anyone can live sweetly, patiently, lovingly, purely, till the sun goes down." How hard can it be to diet for 24 hours *when you know you're going to be able to eat well and be satisfied the following day?*).

If only, I thought, the on-off pattern would prove to be habitual—thereby putting the *subconscious drive* to work *for* me—as I hoped!

I began the diet, determined to combine the two likely extremes of calorie consumption on an every-other-day basis: a "low figure" of 900 or so on one day, my personal "ideal figure" of 3400 on the following.

If things worked out, the 900-day would steadily decrease my fat component while speeding the diet along.

The 3400-day would give me a respite from the previous day's rigors while allowing me to reform my eating habits. (Like a good number of the obese, my custom had been to all but eliminate breakfast, thinking vaguely in terms of "beginning a diet today" when I woke up in the morning. My noontime meal was generally moderate—and I really socked it away in the evening.)

Habit! If it could only prove to be there . . . !

9

The Brief History of a Successful Diet

The simple truth of the matter is: I remained on my new diet for six months and two days—losing a grand total of 61 pounds—*and never broke it even once.*

I had no prescriptions to help me.

I had no doctors supervising my progress (although I did submit to two complete physical examinations—one before and one partway through—just for the record).

I joined no group.

I ate no special foods—or combinations of foods. (That is, I didn't subscribe to the gimmick approaches, stressing one sort over any others. Naturally, on my "dieting day" I attempted to emphasize those which were most nutritious and carried the least amount of calories. On my "eating day" I again ate nutritiously—but with no concern as to whether a particular food was high in calories or not.)

I did not become nervous, irritable or depressed (or any more so than usual, as my family will testify).

I performed no special exercises. (I'm fairly active anyhow, playing a good deal of outdoor basketball and romping with the kids. Though tempted a couple of times, I purposely avoided taking up any additional exercises, therefore being able to isolate the diet itself as the cause of any weight loss.)

I did, however, have a ball.

During those six months I attended eight birthday parties (six of them were within my immediate family), two graduation parties, one Confirmation party (no weddings), and one tenth anniversary class reunion (my wife's). We got together at any number of small get-togethers—whether at our own house or at friends'—and we continued our usual custom of trying to take in a snack and a show at least once a week.

And in every case cited I managed to arrange it so that the event corresponded with my "eating day"—thereby being able to thoroughly enjoy myself with never a hint (aside from my obvious but gradual weight loss) that I was dieting.

This wasn't as difficult a trick as it might first appear. There was some sheer luck involved, of course, insofar as a few of the events were concerned. The six family birthday parties, however, could be scheduled for either the day itself or for the previous evening. Our "weekly night out" alternated easily between Friday and Saturday nights. Casual get-togethers were also easily arranged to correspond with an "eating day." The only real difficulty, in fact, occurred in the last month of the diet when my wife's reunion—important enough to prompt a 600-mile roundtrip—landed on a "diet day." The problem was solved by simply scheduling *two diet days in a row* early in the month, thus rearranging the schedule.

In addition, I found myself enjoying food as I never did before.

Candy to any fat person is a "bad food." Somewhere along the way we're taught it's full of calories and anytime we break down and eat some we're "sinning," thereby earning ourselves a guilty conscience. (Maybe it doesn't make a lot of sense but I think you'll agree that's just about the way it works.)

Well, I found myself enjoying it—with no guilty conscience—for the first time in memory. When you're purposely *trying* to eat 3400 calories in a single day, you soon realize you can't make it on lettuce and chopped liver alone. You need a wide variety of food—and one of the quickest and most enjoyable ways to add on some meaningful calories —without feeling you're stuffing yourself—is through candy.

Naturally, you can only allow yourself so much—but it's such a grand, unfamiliar feeling to be allowed any at all!

Indeed, I found I could actually *keep candy in the house*

(a "first" for me), fill the couple of dishes designed for that purpose—having warned the children that it was for company and daddy only—and still find several pieces remaining a week or a month later!

The same was true of ice cream. My wife would pick up a couple of half-gallons when she went shopping and, despite the love of the entire family for it, there'd still be some remaining the next day—and maybe the day after!

I was learning—through rigid calorie control and habit—to eat so much, enjoy it . . . and no more. This was a lesson I hadn't managed to learn in my entire previous life.

Although there is no way to single out the hour or the day when "habit" actually took over—it's such a gradual, stealthy process—I would say that I was firmly under its influence by the end of the third week. (The three-week period is also cited by others who have completed the diet.)

That is, by the time three weeks had passed, I was fully aware that: 1) This was the easiest and most enjoyable diet I'd ever attempted; 2) I was steadily, gradually and continually losing weight; and 3) *In all probability* I would remain with the diet until my ideal weight was reached, *no matter how long it took*.

This last was a most important consideration.

It would seem that the reason the great majority of the overweight find "quick diets" so attractive is *not* because they have a particular deadline in mind—a wedding, say, or July at the beach. The reason they'd like to be persuaded they can *hurry* through the diet is simply because the process itself is so detestable. They want to get in and get out of it as quickly as possible. It's *less* painful to be hit *once* with a sledgehammer than to have a steady, interminable drop of water splashing between your eyes weeks and months on end (as Chinese torturers are reputed to know). Give a dieter a choice between real agony for a short time and *almost* enough to eat over an extended period and he'll nearly always choose the first (and so would I).

Yet—the principle that "any lasting weight loss takes time" remains as true today as when it was first enunciated. Nutritionists agree it just is not a good idea to attempt to accelerate the process beyond two—two and a half—or *at the very most* three pounds a week.

Prior to the Eating Man's Diet my outlook on any extended program of weight reduction was entirely bleak. Yet I'd learned that the "quick way" was no way to all.

Again let me emphasize, however, that *by the end of the third week* I realized that *in all probability* I would remain with the diet until my ideal weight was reached—*no matter how long it took.*

I had not, obviously, the sensation of one subjected to Chinese water torture.

I did *not* go around feeling progressively hungry (or hungry at all, the great majority of the time).

And it didn't really make much difference to me if I reduced at a steady 10 pounds a month—as I, surprising myself, did*—or cut that figure to only three or four pounds a month.

The point was, I was enjoying myself—and the diet. Obviously I was losing weight—and obviously I would continue to lose as long as I remained faithful to it. In the meantime, I could carry on my normal round of activities with a mind free of thoughts of food, a stomach free of grumbles for food, and a heart free of self-pity because I was "suffering" on a diet!

The program was truly a *breeze,* once those three weeks had passed. With habit behind me, it got progressively easier, an ingrained part of my life—no more difficult to perform than any of the myriad duties we take upon ourselves—getting up and going to bed at certain times, catching certain trains, remembering to be nice to the boss, etc.

Now there were "bad" times as well as "good."

It is not the most pleasant thing in the world to wake up realizing you're only to be allowed 900 calories today—even when you know it's only for one day. It's hardly pleasant in the evening looking forward to nothing solid until breakfast time. (Evenings were always hardest for me—they had so often occasioned my really chowing down. As a personal restriction I therefore forbade myself solids then—whether on the dieting or eating day—except on those occasions

---

* The actual month-by-month breakdown was 17 pounds the first month—*three pounds* the second (as my body adjusted to what was, in good part, a fluid loss) and then *exactly ten pounds each month thereafter.*

when we dined out. It was the most difficult habit to take hold, but take hold it did. I still practice it.)

However, to give you an indication of the relative ease of the program . . . I realized almost immediately that 3400 calories on an eating day amounted to entirely *too much food*. My first 20 days of dieting I kept careful records of everything I ate—but only *estimated* the calories, saving the actual looking them up and writing them down until the following day. Again and again I thought I'd gorged, so unused was I to trying to consume my entire day's ration in a 12-hour period (seven a.m. to seven p.m., say)—I really feared I had gone overboard only to discover that the total would fall somewhere between 2900 and 3100 calories!

Accordingly, after these 20 days I ceased keeping formal track of calories altogether. (This was another thing the initial three-week period did for me: It very clearly indicated "just about how much" I was allowed to eat up to my limit of 3400, thus freeing me of the chore of keeping constant calorie records.) Having fallen well below the limit time and again, I was certain that there was no way I could go over it without *really* knowing about it. So I "settled back" at an average of 3,000 for the entire length of the diet *just making certain* that 1) I did not go over 3400; and 2) that I did not fall below 2600. Even times when I felt no hunger at all —and there were surprisingly many of them—I "forced myself" to eat a big breakfast and a good-sized lunch. Nor would I skimp on supper.

But, as I say, I wound up consuming an average of 400 less calories than I had planned to.

And that was on the eating day.

Now on the diet day, *I also cut down by 400 calories.*

That's right. I averaged only 500 calories per diet day for the six months of the program.

I did this, however, for a very different reason than the eating day cutdown. It wasn't that I wasn't hungry. Obviously, I was sometimes. *But I found it far easier to go hungry on only 500 calories than I did on 900.*

Perhaps it had to do with the fact that—as discussed earlier—it's often so much easier to do *without* than *with*.

I do know that when I consumed the full 900—by absolute limit on that day—there was something about

40

reaching the limit and being unable to go beyond which tended to leave me dissatisfied.

Whereas, when I intentionally cut an already quite abbreviated diet almost in half, the sense of "leeway" gave me a sense of freedom as well. I might feel hungry—*but I didn't feel restricted.*

Interestingly, it wasn't until I'd completed the diet that I learned the full psychological benefits derived from these two approaches. As we'll see in the following chapter, the best way of remaining faithful to the diet is to set a *ceiling* of calories on the diet day (900 is best recommended) contenting yourself to remain below it—and to set *both a ceiling and a floor* on the eating day, neither going above the one nor below the other.

In addition, of course, I was happily aware that I could in no way hurt myself by cutting down to 500 or so calories for *one day*—as opposed to doing it interminably on a less varied diet. To be on the safe side, I'd occasionally take a vitamin-with-iron tablet, but I probably took no more than a dozen of these throughout the course of the program, confident that I was receiving more than adequate nutritional benefit from my on-off combination. (Proper nutrition is no deep, dark mystery; it's actually quite simple to maintain, provided one follows certain basic guidelines—as we'll discuss later.)

One final word about that initial three-week period: The feeling of relative ease and sense of eventual victory that coincided with its termination—as attested to by myself and others—is clearly in line with the usual rule of habit formation. Although it may take six weeks to "lick" an addiction like cigarettes—or longer, perhaps, for other addictions—three weeks is the normal period of probation in the forming of a new habit. It generally takes about three weeks, for instance, for a person to be on a new job before he feels "in the swing of things." Three weeks is the normal time period before an amputee loses the feeling of a "phantom limb." People who undergo cosmetic plastic surgery generally take about three weeks to get used to their new faces.

As I think back to those six months of the diet, I divide them into two distinct periods: the first three weeks when I was still groping, learning, and wondering whether the diet would prove successful or not—and the following five-months-plus when it had become accepted routine, second nature (or perhaps "ten times nature"), and the greater part of my mind and time could be devoted to subjects having nothing whatsoever to do with my weight problem.

The final few weeks of the diet were far easier than the first three, thus clearly indicating that habit—as developed by *finding regular satisfaction in a program of eating that I could indeed carry out over a lifetime* (basically by the eminently simple expedient of dropping the diet day as the six months ended!)—was indeed present and helping things along.

Now it shouldn't be too surprising that there were a host of other psychological factors that helped the program along as well. When things work successfully, there are usually several reasons why—and the Eating Man's Diet is no exception.

Some of these reasons—as advanced by men who should know—are quite fascinating and provide valuable insights into the day-by-day mechanics of the program. I urge you therefore to give them a few moments of your time before we proceed into the quite simple details as to how you may set up your own customized version of the Eating Man's Diet.

10

Some of the Reasons Why

Now we've already seen that habit is a major factor in the working principle of the Eating Man's Diet and that it helps in two ways: 1) by accustoming you to the unavoidable length of a program that calls for a severe weight reduction; and 2) by conditioning you to the acceptance of new eating patterns along the way, so that when the program ends you are prepared to remain at your new weight without the usual urgent desire to recoup your losses.

We've also seen that the diet is absolutely safe (again, let me stress, with your physician's approval) as it is based squarely on the no-gimmick formula of well-rounded, well-balanced meals which you are free to consume on *both days,* as you only actually alternate the *number of calories* (relatively high to relatively low) from one day to the next.

In addition we've seen that the diet is not only nutritionally sound but mathematically sound as well. By alternating high and low calories you tend to lose weight just as if you were consuming the average of the two alternatives (but of course without the feeling of irascibility or persistent hunger that such a program usually entails).

Now as to the additional reasons why it works—let me cite a few experts in the field of psychology.*

* For the record, the comments and opinions of the three psychologists cited in this chapter are in response to my specific request for the same—and should not be interpreted as being based on results

Edward Deaux, Ph.D., of the Behavior Research Laboratory at Antioch College (and acting chairman of the psychology department) says that the diet "actually relies on *several* psychological phenomena" which have been known and studied at length over the past several years "but which have never been applied to anything as useful as a human diet."

Specifically he refers to the "elation" and "depression" effects which were first brought to the attention of the scientific community by L. P. Crespi in 1942 and recently studied under the names Positive-Contrast Effects and Negative-Contrast Effects by Norman Spear of Rutgers.*

What these amazing studies show is that animals will actually respond *more* vigorously when given a certain reward (food, for instance) *"if on alternate trials they are given a smaller amount."* (!)

When the subject is consistently given the same size reward—despite the fact that it be the equivalent of the larger size in the first instance—his performance is measurably less vigorous.

The comparison of these two reactions, says Deaux, "bears out much the same effect that your diet relies on."

In other words, it would seem that the previously mentioned phenomenon of the 3400-calorie day as being entirely too much to eat is at least partially based on what Crespi and Spears discovered. Prior to my beginning the diet I

---

they themselves have obtained. One of them, however (I will not say which), has actually applied the principles of the Eating Man's Diet to his personal weight problem with seemingly very satisfactory results. Having had considerable difficulty in stabilizing his weight following a severe diet (which he undertook before learning of the Eating Man's Diet and on which he lost a total of 46 pounds), he began utilizing the EMD principle to such success that he recently wrote me that he had managed to gain not a single pound while *not* keeping track of his calories but simply relying on "the habits that have been established . . . in spite of a week's vacation eating in New Orleans!!" The double exclamation point in the quote is indeed his, by the way, but a good deal of the *emphasis* in this chapter's quotes (in the form of italics) is mine, rather than that of the original authors.

* L. P. Crespi, American Journal of Psychology, 55, 467, 1942; L. P. Crespi, Psychological Review, 51, 341, 1944; N. E. Spear and J. H. Spitzner, Psychological Monographs: General and Applied, 80, 1966 (No. 10)

would have undoubtedly found 3400 not too much at all—since it can be seen that in order to sustain my 230-pound weight I most probably averaged between 3400 and 4600 calories.

However, the *contrast* between 3400 and 900 (or 3000 and 500) was so great that the larger number of calories seemed quite a magnificent "reward" preceding and following the abbreviated number. We all are subject to such contrasts—as today's grammar school scientists know. One of the first experiments children usually are given is the one involving three pans of water—one hot, one cold and one lukewarm. After holding the left hand in the hot water and the right hand in the cold water for a couple of minutes, they then put both hands into the lukewarm and are surprised to find that their left hand tells them it's "cold" while their right hand says it's "hot."

The larger number of calories seems a real reward despite the fact that it might possibly be considerably below what your usual average is. The contrast makes all the difference.

Now James H. Elder, Ph.D., recently retired from the psychology department of Washington State University, also stresses the reward aspect of the diet, noting that "the only substantial reinforcement or reward one gets from following a *regular* schedule of self-denial comes from scale readings of weight loss. These changes may be rather small and not sufficient to maintain motivation for adhering to a rigid day-after-day program of restraint *which in itself is rather punishing.*

"The Eating Man's Diet, on the other hand, provides *regular daily reinforcement* (i.e., reward). *A person following the program gets the usual satisfaction from food on his 'eating days' and, on low calorie days, the reward of having succeeded in following the schedule.*"

Dr. Elder thus accounts for the relative ease of *both* days. Unlike the animals in Crespi's studies, human beings are able to derive particular satisfaction from the "short end" as well as the larger one. You could say it's "only" an intellectual or emotional satisfaction—but coupled with the physical satisfaction of the following day, it totals up to a *most satisfying program.*

"The chief advantages over most diet schedules," continues Dr. Elder, "should be the periodic reinforcements and the relative absence of aversive stimulation. Most dietary programs demand constant vigilance and continuous voluntary inhibition of eating responses. Any diet which requires constant restraint *increases the probability of deviations or exceptions*. These, in turn, may produce guilt reactions and lower motivation for getting back on the schedule."

Break a regular diet and, as you well know, it's murder to begin again. One gets the feeling he has dropped a carefully wound ball of string and the only way to resume winding it is to start back at the beginning—a most dreaded task.

But the Eating Man's Diet, by virtue of its built-in breaks, practically eliminates the "guilt reactions" Dr. Elder cites and on the occasions when it *must* be broken has proven to be quite easily resumed. (One 62-year-old woman, for instance, who proclaims that she had "never before" been able to stick to a diet, happened to come down with a rather severe cold just a month after beginning this one. Wisely she dropped the diet for a week while recuperating. But at the end of the week, feeling fine, *she immediately resumed the diet,* remained on it *six more months,* losing at the specially devised rate of a pound a week, *and retains her total loss of 31 pounds to this date.*)

"Another feature of the Eating Man's Diet," Dr. Elder concludes, "is that the schedule is *consistent with the facts relating to established habit patterns*. The objective here seems quite similar, and no more difficult, than adaptation to work or class schedules which require rising at earlier hours on alternate days. *This is accomplished by millions of people with a few weeks of practice.* The daily routine involved in the Eating Man's Diet seems to be quite consistent with well-established principles of psychology."

("—a few weeks of practice," Dr. Elder says, happily stressing that point. Remember, even though the diet *may* seem initially easy to you, *habit will not form overnight.* It *will* form after "a few weeks of practice.")

Professor William Verplanck of the University of Tennessee introduces a couple of factors which hadn't occurred to me at all, one of them clearly explaining the importance of having a *floor* (that is, a minimum amount of calories) as well as a *ceiling* (a maximum amount) on the eating day.

"The requirement that the dieter consume *his full quotient* of calories (on the eating day) is a very sound method for the development of the desired eating habits. It means that on *some* occasions he will need to eat more than he *needs* to, which is unpleasant—and *unpleasant it should be to eat more than required.*"

As pointed out, other dieters and I were often tempted to *undereat* on that day, so strong were we—and often not at all hungry—after weeks or months on the diet. But we stuck to the on-off principle, *eating even though at times it seemed unpleasant.* (That big, big breakfast, which I often delighted in, *was* hard getting down sometimes—especially on those occasional mornings when I'd gotten a late start.) But, here— talk about habit formation!—the diet was teaching me, for the first time in my life, that eating food under obligation *can* be no fun at all. For the first time I was able to see the point of view of those scores of people I've sat opposite from in restaurants, school cafeterias and army mess halls who— well-prepared food or not—"just didn't feel like eating." No longer did food seem to me a be-all, end-all and cure-all.

(Perhaps the best day of my diet, in fact—the day I absolutely knew I was going to make it—occurred about halfway into the program. The previous day, an eating day, had been one of those where everything *really* goes wrong. From mid-afternoon on, things got blacker and blacker. At home that night I took my wife's head off for some inconsequential trifle and when I went to bed, still upset, it was a good while before I fell asleep. The very special thing about that day never dawned on me until the following morning. In much better spirits by then, I had the sudden realization that, as bad as things had seemed to get—*it had never once entered my mind to try to solve my problem by overeating!* In fact, I had barely hit the minimum of 2600 calories for the day. *Food just didn't appeal to me.* This was, of course, the reverse of every experience with food that I remembered. From that day forward I ceased to raise the *possibility* of failure, thanks—at least in part—to the fact that I had learned that eating *could* be unpleasant, however empty the stomach and well-prepared the food.)

Professor Verplanck also points out that the very *irregularity* of the diet—on again, off again—prevents one from falling into the rut of simple acceptance of his food and forces him to *think about what he's eating.*

"Having both on and off days requires the dieter to give a good deal of thought to *exactly* what he eats," says Professor Verplanck. "This is optimal for learning *about* food, and to eat it *thoughtfully* . . . which is what fat people need to do."

(One woman, who had become quite adept at counting calories long before beginning this diet, told me how strange it seemed to her to sit down to an 800 or 900 calorie meal and intentionally total up items such as buttered sweet potatoes, custard pudding and an after-dinner liqueur. She said she'd been accustomed to keeping track of calories only when the meal totaled 400 or 500. Anything beyond that, she said, and "it just didn't seem like dieting . . . So why bother to count?" She realizes now that refusing to count beyond 500 was one of the principal reasons she'd originally gained weight.)

Now I'd like to offer just a couple of more thoughts on the diet before bringing this chapter to a close. Feel free to skip them if you wish and go on to the next chapter. I only present them here because—as you'll find, should you attempt the diet yourself—it works so all but miraculously well (indeed, at least one woman who went on it says she really thinks it *is* a miracle) a certain fascination about its mysteries develops as you remain on it. *Why*, you continue to ask yourself, *am I so able to lose weight now—when I never could before?* You'll find yourself, I'm sure, discovering fresh insights into it regularly. Such has been the experience of those who have already succeeded with it.

The first thought has to do with the "ghost appetite," which we discussed before. Just why is it that that appetite—feeling you need to eat even though it can be "shown" you are not physiologically hungry—is not readily aroused by this method?

Well, my own conclusion is that this mechanism within us, whatever it consists of, is only triggered by a *prolonged* program of reduction. Seeming to "end" the diet every other day, you satisfy your immediate hunger and your body does not build up this seeming *backlog* of hunger. The mechanism seems quite similar to that which controls your sleep needs. You *can* go without sleep for a good deal of time, operating on what is commonly called "nervous energy." However, when at last sleep comes, the backlog of lack of sleep can hit you really hard, and cause you to be tired for days on end. If, on the other hand, you intermittently satisfy your sleep requirement with catnaps—as Edison, for instance, did—you may continue working for as long or longer than the one who subsists on nervous energy—but the backlog never really hits you. By continually satisfying your sleep—or food—requirement before it becomes too pronounced, you prevent the buildup that might later cause an "explosion."

Now Verplanck would also seem to take note of this phenomenon—but in a different manner. He refers to Schacter's studies, which clearly demonstrate that the obese tend to have a far different response to physiological hunger than do the normal. (Normal people tend to base their desire for food on "internal cues"—i.e., physiological hunger—whereas the obese often base theirs on external cues: the time of day, the smell of a frying steak, the sight of a banana split, etc.) "A necessary condition for a subject to learn to discriminate his state of nutrition on the basis of internal cues, rather than of external ones," he says, "is to provide the subject with the appropriate stable internal cues regularly. This stability is provided nicely by your (eating) days."

This desire to eat when full—although occasioned by outside stimuli—is what I call "ghost appetite." In any case, the diet helps to control it—and in completing the diet, you banish this unreasonable hunger.

The second—and final—thought before we proceed to *your* program has to do with the modern wonder of self-image psychology.

As Maxwell Maltz, M.D., F.I.C.S., points out in his excellent book *Psycho-Cybernetics,** there has been relatively little written on the subject, not because it hasn't worked "but because it has worked so amazingly well." The results in particular cases challenge credibility—and if you haven't read the book, I urge you to.

Now one of self-image psychology's basic tenets is that if you are to *become* a particular sort of person, you must

* Published by Prentice-Hall, Inc., Englewood Cliffs, N. J.

begin to act as if you were *already* that sort of person *now*. (It is *not* necessary that you act that way "fulltime"—at first. But it is recommended that you have regular practice periods which—through *habituating yourself* to react in certain patterns—help bring the transition about.)

I know of no diet that guarantees you can be thin tomorrow.

But the Eating Man's Diet allows you to *react* just as if you were thin tomorrow!

The fact that you can actually "think thin" and continually practice "acting thin" is in no small measure, I'm sure, responsible for its success.

There are, of course, several diets available today—low calorie ones—which tell you you can eat all you please, providing that "all you please" consists of next-to-no-calorie green vegetables, clear bouillon and sugarless carbonated beverages.

Indeed, some of these diets actually recommend you start stuffing yourself with asparagus spears—right out of the can —if you begin to feel "an irresistible urge" to have, say, a chocolate bonbon.

Now this may be great for your figure—at that particular moment—but I can't help but wonder what it does to your self-image. Aside from the immediate calorie consideration, is that furtive figure sitting in a semi-darkened kitchen— opening and devouring one can of asparagus after another— really so far removed from one who raids the icebox and bites into some honest-to-goodness, satisfying *food?*

But to go ahead and *have* a chocolate bonbon when you want a chocolate bonbon! And to do it just like your slim "eat-anything-she-likes" friend who *instinctively* knows her limit is three (whereas, at first, you'll have to rely on totaling calories to tell you this)—you begin almost at once to associate yourself mentally with those who eat well and eat *successfully,* rather than the poor "glutton" who is so anxious to fill her mouth with *something* she'll settle for asparagus spears—or even cotton wadding.

And again, we're not talking about six months from now or a year from now or two months from now—when you've completed your diet. We're talking about *tomorrow*. Immediately.

That's how soon you can start.

In a very real sense—in a mental and emotional one—you actually can be *thin* as soon as tomorrow!

And, as the days pass, and you eventually become *physically* thin as well, you'll have all that mental and emotional background on tap and ready to *keep* you there.

Eat well tonight if you like. Enjoy yourself. Because, *if you make the decision,* you'll have a long, long time ahead of you to *continue* enjoying yourself—and your food—and your newfound slimness.

Starting as soon as tomorrow . . .

11

Your Own Diet— Custom-Made

The actual mechanics of setting up your own customized version of the Eating Man's Diet are quite simple.

Having received your physician's approval to diet, you need only follow the three steps described below. (Do not, however, begin your program until you've read the final chapter *carefully*.)

1. Consult Chart A in the appendix and, depending on your sex, height and general body build, determine your ideal weight *range*—and then, at your discretion, a number within that range which is most likely to be your ideal weight. (If the range, for instance, is 123 to 138 pounds, you might well choose the midpoint figure: 130.)

2. Apply this figure to Chart B—which contains the minimum and maximum number of calories you are to be allowed on your eating day, plus the "Diet Ideal": the figure between these two extremes *which you should consistently aim at*.

3. Begin the regular alternation of this number of calories with *a maximum of 900 calories on your diet day*.

Yes, that's all there is to it.

Now you may well wonder: *How much will I lose weekly on the Eating Man's Diet? How long will the entire process take?*

The answer depends on several factors—and is probably best arrived at by way of an example.

Let's say, for instance, you're a woman of medium frame, 5'6" tall whose present weight is 165 pounds.

By consulting Chart A you determine your ideal weight is between 123 and 138 pounds . . . or, taking the midpoint, 130.

Now by consulting Chart B you see you should therefore consume a minimum of 1950 calories, a maximum of 2600 calories and a Diet Ideal of 2300.

You then begin to alternate 2300 calories regularly with 900.

The amount of weight you lose weekly will depend on how close the Diet Ideal is to the actual ideal.

That is, the number of calories you're allowed to consume on your eating day *should* match the actual number you would normally "burn" on that day—just as closely as possible. But until you actually arrive at your ideal weight and begin to regularly maintain that weight, there is no sure way of telling what your *exact* number of maintenance calories is.

Remember, the minimum and maximum number of calories allowed you on your eating day have been determined by multiplying your ideal weight by 15 (for those who are relatively inactive) and by 20 (for those who are quite active). The Diet Ideal (the midpoint figure—rounded off by no more than 25 calories) indicates average activity, a quite suitable figure for the great majority of us.

Now, assuming that your activity *is* actually average, and that you would ordinarily burn off 2300 calories daily, you will therefore lose approximately two pounds weekly for the length of the diet. Since you have a total of 35 pounds to lose, it'll take you about 17 weeks—or four months—to arrive at 130 pounds.

Loss of weight at this rate is fine—and very close to the ideal. However, you can see that if your activity is consistently above average, you may find yourself losing at 2½ pounds per week. If it is consistently below average, you may only lose 1½ pounds per week. Either of these figures, however, is suitable. In the first case, you would arrive at your goal in 14 weeks; in the second it would take about 23 weeks.

At this point, having arrived at your ideal weight, you may then drop the 900-calorie day and continue at your Diet

Ideal number of calories on a daily basis. If your weight remains stable—you do not gain or lose—you'll know your Diet Ideal and *actual ideal* are the same thing and you can quite simply—and easily—continue consuming calories at that rate.

If, however, you should continue to lose some weight, it is because the Diet Ideal is actually a little low for your normal activity. By gradually increasing the number of calories you consume in a 24-hour period—at increments of, say, 50 to 100—you'll soon find your actual ideal calorie consumption and, with a little practice, will be able to eat that much regularly.

If, on the other hand, you find yourself beginning to gain some weight back after dropping the 900-calorie day, it *may* be because your Diet Ideal is set a bit high for your normal activity—*or it may be because your body is making a final water adjustment.*

In either case, don't panic.

Simply resume the Eating Man's Diet as before, dropping to 900 calories *for one day* and then resuming your Diet Ideal consumption.

Do not attempt to eat at the rate of 900 calories more than one day without breaking for your Diet Ideal day—and do not attempt to immediately lower the number of calories you consume on your Diet Ideal day.

Bear in mind that your Diet Ideal and actual ideal *may* be the same thing and you've only a water adjustment to wait out.

Now throughout this book we have referred to the vagaries of water adjustment: the fact that you may seem to be losing weight while only losing water—and the fact that you may actually be losing weight, but because you are *not* losing water the loss will not show up on your scale.

How do you tell the difference between the real gain or loss and the false gain or loss?

There is only one way: and that is through time.

Fortunately, the Eating Man's Diet is *less* susceptible to these vagaries than are other diets because of its alternate-day nature, That is, you may find yourself "losing" three pounds on a 900-calorie day and "gaining back" *almost* three pounds on an eating day, indicating that the water balance is fairly constant *after each eating day* and weighing yourself after an eating day will give you a fairly accurate picture of what your actual weight is. (On another diet— without constant breaks—you might believe you'd lost a certain amount of weight, resume eating normally and find you hadn't actually come within ten pounds of that hoped-for loss.) But even the Eating Man's Diet cannot entirely overcome the water problem. At what might seem to be the diet's end, you may find you still have an *actual loss* of two or three pounds to go. Therefore I strongly suggest you do not tamper with the Diet Ideal number of calories (if you seem to gain a little weight back) until you have continued on the plan for two more weeks.

If, with two weeks passed, you still seem to edge up a little over your ideal weight, *slightly modify* your Diet Ideal by 50 or 100 calories (while continuing to alternate with 900-calorie days) until your weight remains stable at its ideal.

Most probably at the end of your diet, you'll find yourself *gradually* eliminating the 900-calorie day. In other words, instead of a straight alternation of eating and diet days, you'll begin to have two eating days in a row—then three—then four—then a whole week's worth of eating days without the necessity of introducing a diet day. Eventually, of course, you'll do away with the diet day altogether—*but keeping it in reserve should your weight ever again begin to climb.*

You'll find it quite simple to introduce a diet•day if your weight climbs a pound above your ideal—and the very introduction of that day will serve to remind you of the habits you worked so hard to establish, enabling you to resume them once more. Thus, when at last you reach your ideal weight, you can be perfectly confident that you will stay there.

Another question you might raise is: *What happens if I lose at less than the rate of 1½ pounds per week?*

The answer to this one depends on you.

If after three or four weeks of the diet—with your initial loss well out of the way—you find yourself only averaging a pound a week, say, you may do one of two things:

The first is to adjust your food consumption on either your diet day, eating day, or both days. You may find, for instance, that you prefer continuing to consume the number of calories you already *are* consuming on your eating day and choose to cut your diet day by 200 or 300 calories. Such a decrease will not hurt you—since you are consuming those few calories only on an alternate-day basis. However, towards the diet's end, you may find yourself having to cut into the Diet Ideal number of calories anyway, in order to arrive at your true maintenance figure.

Therefore, it would probably be wiser to cut into the Diet Ideal number. Go ahead, if you like—*but do not in any case cut it beneath the stipulated eating day minimum.*

Remember, unless you have a definite *floor* on the number of calories you consume that day—your minimum as determined by multiplying your ideal weight by 15—you are merely *undereating on both days* and thereby nullifying the entire principle of the diet. Certainly it's conceivable that you may be anxious to lose weight and therefore wish to be as harsh on yourself on the two days as you possibly can. However, if your anxiety is such that you will not follow the principle of the diet—that you will refuse to satisfy your desire for food—you'll accomplish no more than a short-lived weight loss followed by a rapid return to your original status. *I cannot overemphasize that you should in no case seek to consume less than the minimum number of calories called for on the eating day.* Only by consuming that number with regularity will you build up habit . . . which is, of course, what this diet—and your eating problem—are basically about.

Now I said you could do one of *two* things if you find yourself losing only a pound or so a week.

The second approach—and one which a surprising percentage of those who have successfully completed the diet decided to take—is just to sit back, relax and enjoy it.

By the time you're on the Eating Man's Diet three or four weeks, after all, habit and the relative ease of the diet will be very much with you. One woman, for instance, who had only 22 pounds to lose, *took just over five months to lose them*. By choice. She says it was very clear to her by the time one month had passed that the weight was quite gradually disappearing and—since she was not that much overweight to start with—she found herself in no hurry. Besides, she said she'd never enjoyed a diet so much before. As long as she "didn't *feel* like (she) was dieting," and as long as the weight was nonetheless coming off, she figured: "Why bother to speed things up?" *This woman had been trying one diet after another for four years without success.* Yet today she has no trouble maintaining her weight loss.

All right. I understand the minimum number and the Diet Ideal. What about the maximum number of calories? How free should I feel to consistently hit that maximum?

Feel perfectly free to consistently hit the maximum—as long as you are consistently losing at the rate of *at least one pound per week*—and as long as this rate of loss is satisfactory to you.

In the case where you're *not* losing at a pound a week— or *are,* but wish to lose *more*—you should naturally drop to the vicinity of the Diet Ideal.

But again, if the weight is consistently coming off and you are personally satisfied with your progress, stay with the maximum if you like. *Just don't go over it.*

Not going over the maximum is quite as important as *not going under* the minimum.

It *is* possible, of course, that you will actually lose weight consistently going over the maximum because of the severity of your diet day.

But, as with going under the minimum, you are nullifying the purpose of the diet. This is *not*—repeat, *not*—a method in which you are allowed to "starve and stuff." The purpose of the eating day is in no way associated with the dieter's stuffing himself. The purpose is to allow you a pleasant respite from the diet day restrictions—while you adapt yourself to habits of eating which are designed to last you a lifetime.

If you consistently go over the maximum, *that* will be your habit. And when at last you quit the diet day itself, your weight will steadily come back on.

Again, as pointed out in the beginning of this chapter, the Diet Ideal is *"the midpoint figure that you should consistently aim at."*

Most probably you'll find—as most of us have—that trying to consume the maximum number of calories each day is too much, while trying to consume the minimum is just not as satisfying.

Aim at the middle. *Aim* at the Diet Ideal. You have wide

latitude on either side and should you miss dead center, don't worry about it. *But do keep aiming.*

A principal advantage of this wide latitude is that you are freed from the often disagreeable task of having to keep a running calorie count. (If you're aiming right at the maximum and your mate brings home some super special dessert for supper, what do you do? Either settle for the one you'd planned—or break your diet. If you've figured steak for supper will bring you up to the exact maximum—and you wind up having ham or corned beef instead, does that mean you'll go over or under your maximum figure? Or won't you have to whip out the old calorie counter in order to really know for sure?)

When you aim at the Diet Ideal with patient regularity, it doesn't take long at all to determine *approximately* the amount of food you're allowed on an eating day. And therefore you are pretty well able to standardize your meals (something we all tend to do anyway)—but by *type of food* rather than precise calorie count.

In other words, you may find the Diet Ideal number of calories allows you to have a gelatin dessert with a couple of tablespoons of whipped cream with your noon meal. Well, if you like gelatin desserts, this is just fine—but one day there may be a special on strawberry pie and you may decide to order the pie instead. So you consciously "make room for it" (as your eat-anything-she-likes friend unconsciously does) by eliminating a piece of bread and butter with your meal.

The question is: *Can you afford the extra calories?*

Well, here's what you've actually done: You've substituted a 375-calorie dessert for 325 calories worth of gelatin, whipped cream, bread and butter—a 50-calorie surplus.

The answer to *can you afford an extra 50 calories?* is definitely *yes.* And you don't have to write them down, take them home and add them up.

Remember: Throughout the Eating Man's Diet you are consciously training yourself to eat in the same manner all normally slim people eat. The "leeway" you have allowed yourself by consistently *aiming at* the Diet Ideal is ample to cover an extra 50, 100 or 200 calories *now and then.* By the time you've completed three weeks of the diet, you *should* know exactly what you are allowed for breakfast each morning (since breakfast is the most consistent of all meals), and approximately what you are allowed for lunch and supper (is it one potato?, two potatoes?, bread *and* potatoes?, no potatoes but an extra serving of meat?, can you eat dessert after *both* meals or only *one* meal?, etc.). Knowledge of this sort is far more important than knowing what the calorie difference is between butter and margarine,* boiled and baked potatoes,** or baked and broiled bluefish.***

By knowing you are allowed an "average serving" of meat for supper, the leeway in your diet will allow you to freely substitute barbecued beef (300) for boiled beef (250) or beef stroganoff (350) or even beef stew (250). Similarly, you might have lamb stew (250), chicken chop suey (275), pork chop suey (300) or a couple of frankfurters (250).

All of these are within the same general range.

The fact that you realize you're allowed one "average serving" of meat for approximately 300 calories will make exact totals unnecessary.

Naturally, you should be aware that the addition of such extras as breading or certain types of gravy can really multiply the calories—and that average servings of some meats are really quite low (three slices of lean bacon, for instance, total only 120 calories).

However, by keeping the Diet Ideal constantly in mind—and by purposely checking on your calorie consumption every so often in order to "keep yourself honest"—you'll find that in time you'll quite naturally skip your luncheon dessert on a day when you have an unscheduled jelly doughnut at your coffee break—or you'll content yourself with salad and broth for supper on an evening when you and your best guy or girl plan to go out for pizza and beer.

How many times have you heard others (or yourself) say: "Well, I'm off my diet tonight. I simply can't pass up that (*you fill in the blank:* pecan pie?, ice cream?, a special flaming dessert?)." During the Eating Man's Diet—and later, when the formal diet itself is over—you won't pass up that (*fill in the blank*) either, *but neither will it ever put an ounce of weight on you.*

* No difference. A pat of either is 50 calories.
** 20 calories. One medium baked is 100; one medium boiled is 80.
*** 15 calories. Bluefish baked is 200; bluefish broiled is 185.

59

12

Some Additional Questions

Because of the particular nature of the Eating Man's Diet—its placing the final responsibility for the fashioning of your personal program upon your own shoulders, rather than insisting you follow strict doctrinaire imperatives on a cut-and-dried daily regimen (as most diets must!)—it necessarily provokes a host of questions. These in turn, because of the vast spectrum of individual dieters, cannot be given simple *yes or no* answers.

Accordingly, this and the following chapter will be devoted to those questions which have actually arisen in the past and are most likely to arise again in the future. Most probably, a few of them have already occurred to *you:*

The variations in calories allowed for on the "eating day" schedule seem clear. But what about on the "diet day"? How harsh may I be on myself then?

Just as harsh as you'd like—provided that your constitution will let you get away with it. It makes little sense, I'm sure you realize, to intentionally set out to have *zero* calories on your diet day, suffer through this regimen two or three times and then blow the diet sky-high. Moderation is necessarily called for—especially during the diet's initial three-week period.

The best method on the 900-calorie day is to carefully plan three 300-calorie meals (or three 250-calorie meals and a late 150-calorie snack) and either consume the calories or "eliminate" them as you go.

That is, you want to beware of putting your calories aside during the day and saving them for a grand eating binge in the evening. If you schedule a 300-calorie breakfast but eat only 100 calories instead, you should regard those extra 200 calories as gone, lost, irretrievable—*not* something to be applied on your evening meal.

Of course, the *main point* is to consume no more than 900 calories on your diet day—and on occasion a trade off of morning for evening calories *may* be justified. I caution you against making a practice of it, however, both because it approaches the starve-and-binge-eat syndrome so often associated with the obese, and because food is more satisfying when taken *early*—as a *prevention* for hunger, than *late*— as a *cure*.

The simple truth is, you are far less likely to overeat in the evening if you make yourself consume a suitable breakfast and lunch. Thankfully, you *will* have less trouble consuming a big breakfast on your eating day than you may have had in the past due to the fact that a diet day immediately precedes it.

On your diet day, however, your best approach remains to begin it with the idea of eating your full quota of 900 calories, and then—should you decide to try to get by on less—do not compensate your undereating at particular meals with your overeating at others.

All right, getting back to the eating day . . . I notice your own diet stressed a "big, big breakfast" and no solids after supper. Are we expected to eat in the same manner?

Not at all. In the appendix you'll find representative eating day menus for allowable calorie consumptions ranging from 1600 to 3500 calories per day. You'll note that the number of meals on these menus vary between three and six (!)—the latter allowing you "coffee-and" breaks in the morning and afternoon and a late night snack in addition to your three regular meals.

A weightwatching group I briefly joined a few years back (with, as in the case of so many attempts I made, no successful results) had as a principle what still seems to me a rather sound idea: Find out what area of eating your problem lies in—and *attack that area.*

If you're relatively untroubled by a tendency to late night

snacking and its hand-in-hand corollary: skipping breakfast in the morning—there is no real reason to eliminate a late night snack from your diet.

If on the other hand you find, as I have found in the past, that a few extra calories after supper trigger your appetite to have a few *more*—and a few *more*—you're wise to eat defensively: Take on an ounce of prevention early rather than a pound of cure later.

"Breakfast like a king, lunch like a prince and supper like a pauper" is a method of eating that pays great dividends. A good-sized breakfast (not necessarily "a big, big one") tends —or *seems*—to remain with you throughout the day, constantly warding off hunger and helping you to fight temptations as they arise.

In any case, choice of the size of your breakfast is entirely yours. Just remember that however you decide to divide up your meals on your eating day, you are now establishing the habits that are to remain with you for a lifetime. *The more sensible your daily menu is now, the better it will serve you later.*

Earlier in this book you mentioned group diets as being "preferable," in your opinion, to any aside from the Eating Man's Diet. I was wondering: Might it be possible for me to continue meeting with my group while practicing the Eating Man's Diet principles?

Certainly—depending on the sort of group you belong to.

There are some groups, of course, which jealously insist upon their own brand of reducing programs—which, of course, is their right. Obviously, however, it would be impractical for you to belong to such a group while attempting to follow a different method of dieting.

Other groups, however, allow the choice of diet to be squarely up to you (or your doctor). There is no reason you could not meet with such a group as an added incentive to help you along in your program. (Similarly, there is no reason why you cannot follow the Eating Man's Diet under a cooperating doctor's direct supervision—if you like.) The only danger—a seemingly minor one—is that you may develop a dependence on the group and be unable to "go it alone" later.

At any rate, I would strongly advise you *not* to enter into a group situation until you have completed at least three weeks of the Eating Man's Diet and the habit principle has begun to take hold. Group members tend to exchange both recipes and diet theories and you might be persuaded to tamper with the principle prior to the passage of that initial period—neither more nor less so than with any other diet. As you'll see in the final chapter, it is *most* important that those three weeks run smooth and successful. If a breakdown in the program is going to occur, it will most probably occur *then*. With the three weeks completed, however, you *won't* be talked out of the diet and you undoubtedly *will* make converts!

I've been looking at the menus in the back of the book. I see you're not at all hesitant to recommend "empty calories"—those foods which have relatively small food values as compared with their caloric content. Am I not really better off trying to eliminate these calories as much as possible —and stress such things as meats, vegetables, milk, etc.?

On another diet—yes. On the Eating Man's Diet—no.

Again, you must bear in mind that what you are trying to accomplish on your eating day is to eat as closely as possible to the manner in which you hope to *continue* eating when the diet is ended. Stressing the generally accepted highly nutritional food is good—*but not to the exclusion of all other types*.

Now if you're opposed, as some people are, to sugar products, wheat products, meat products or dairy products—and have no intention of consuming these things when the diet is ended, naturally you will not wish to consume them while *on* the diet either. (The same goes for alcoholic products, by the way.) Fine. The menus in the back are *merely suggested,* after all, as an aid to helping you determine menus of your own. Feel free to dismiss them entirely, if you wish.

However, if you *do* intend to eat ice cream again—or bread and butter, chocolate candy, meat and potatoes—if you intend to have an occasional drink—it's *absolutely necessary* that your eating patterns while on the diet reflect those eventualities.

If your "sweet tooth" is such, for instance, that you go absolutely mad for Scottish short bread or salt water taffy— and have no intention of altogether eliminating this sweet nuisance from your life—the time to practice adapting yourself to its consumption *within limits* is during the Eating Man's Diet itself, not afterwards when your weight and resolve (and guard) are down. Too often the end of a diet signals a *carte blanche* return to "freedom" and old habits. Practice allowing yourself "limited freedom" now—and you'll have that habit the rest of your life.

Other diets have as their *only concern* removing weight from you as mathematically quickly as possible, and to consume "empty calories" *intentionally* while on them is, of course, inappropriate. Such, however, is not the case with the Eating Man's Diet.

Now I've stressed the word *"intentionally"* because—as you'll recall in the Introduction—I stated that empty calories were *"absolutely essential*—assuming normal health—to the dieter who was determined to achieve and sustain his ideal weight."

Well, I'm sure you see by now that I base this conclusion —at least in part—on the habit principle of the diet.

However, there is a sound nutritional basis as well. The fact of the matter is: If your eating habits are, in general, nutritionally correct, it takes *extremely little food* to provide all of your main food requirements—aside from calories themselves—in a particular period.

Your body, seemingly "aware" of its vast and continuing need for calories, uses itself as a storehouse for them. However, the provision it makes for the other needs nutritionists are forever emphasizing are considerably less—as it tends to accept only those proteins, vitamins, minerals, etc. that it can *immediately* use—rejecting any surplus as if it were poison. (Indeed, people—children especially—*have been poisoned* through continuing overdoses of vitamin pills.) The fact that a little of these food values is good for you just does not lead to the conclusion that a lot are *very* good for you.

Does this mean nutritionists are somehow mistaken in emphasizing these food values? Not at all. The very fact that the body consistently eliminates all surplus demonstrates why regular intake is highly advisable. In most cases an "overdose" will not hurt you a bit. My point is, however, it will not *help* you either.

Once you've "stocked up" on those values your body has

an immediate need for, anything over and above that re quirement—whether in the form of beefsteak, green vegetables or sugar-coated vitamin pills—becomes in effect "empty calories" anyway. That is, it does no more real good in your system than an ice cream cone or a piece of pie.

The nutritional basis for my saying empty calories are "absolutely essential" is that they are, quite simply, unavoidable. To give you an idea of how very little your minimal requirements are—suppose you, a normally healthy man or woman, sit down for breakfast one morning to *three tablespoons of peanut butter, one-half orange* and *one multiple vitamin-with-iron pill.* From that point on, any calories you consume will, in effect, be empty!

For you've taken care of your protein, calcium, iron, vitamin A, thiamine, riboflavin and niacin (vitamin B complex), ascorbic acid (vitamin C) and vitamin D—all those necessities (aside from such things as fat, water and certain minute "trace" requirements) that have been determined as minimally necessary to proper nutrition.

This does not, of course, mean that I advocate such a patently unappealing breakfast or approach to nutritional satisfaction.

The best approach to nutrition for the normally healthy is the regular consumption of meat, fish, eggs, milk, fruit, vegetables and starches. Once you've had your "minimums" of these foods (as listed in the appendix), you may feel free to enjoy your limit of calories in whatever form is most pleasing to you.

Meat? Eggs? Milk? But what about cholesterol? As long as we're "practicing habits" designed to remain with us the rest of our lives, isn't this a good time to begin cutting down on this substance which is often singled out as a factor in heart disease?

As I write, there has as yet been no "causative link" established between cholesterol consumption and heart disease. Many nutritionists, in fact, deny that such a link exists.

However, there is an increasing body of evidence that the relationship may indeed be causative and if you wish to keep your cholesterol consumption down "just to be on the safe side," there's certainly no reason you cannot do so while on the Eating Man's Diet.

But I should point out to you that a complete elimination

of cholesterol is neither recommended nor feasible. Often you can bring your daily consumption within recommended limits by doing no more than substituting polyunsaturated margarine and polyunsaturated cooking oil for the butter and animal fat you may be presently using. Seeing to it that your beef is lean puts it in the same cholesteral range as that of fresh fish. Drinking skimmed milk instead of whole also dramatically cuts down on cholesterol.

Just don't make the mistake of assuming—as some do—that high-calorie foods are in any way equated with those which are high in cholesterol. Pizza, for instance, has little cholesterol itself. The meat that decorates it, however, may be high. To cut down on your cholesterol intake you can order it plain—or with a mushroom topping. Ice cream is only medium in cholesterol. Hard candy and beer have none!

Eggs—or, more properly, egg yolks—*are* high, but that's only relatively speaking. The amount of cholesterol in a little egg yolk (the whites have none) should not be harmful to you, especially if you make a practice of otherwise reducing your consumption as described above.

One of the Eating Man's Diet's more interesting features, by the way, is that rather than recommend or discourage certain foods—which other diets, by their natures, *must* do—it instead advocates a *system of eating,* a handy umbrella, as it were, that easily covers a multiple of diets. If your desire is a low-cholesterol diet—or if you'd prefer to choose recipes and menus for your 900-calorie days from the literally thousands of low-calorie agendas that have been published in the last several years, ignore those *suggested* in the back. *Just follow the system!*

One thing bothers me. I realize that in order to deal with the widest possible audience you have applied the "rule of thumb" method (15 or 20 times the body weight) in order to set minimums and maximums on eating day calorie consumption. However, in my case I KNOW my normal activity is especially full. Wouldn't it be wiser for me therefore to take the maximum figure you offer as my Diet Ideal since it's probably closer to the true number of calories I burn in a single day?

Actually, no—not in the diet's initial three weeks.

Nutritionists have widely different ideas on how many

calories "should" be allowed to sustain different body weights, some of the top nutritionists freely contradicting others.

I've used the "rule of thumb" method here simply because of its wide latitude. The truth is, individual requirements vary sharply—and the only way you'll be able to determine what your *actual ideal* is will be through your own experience both on the diet itself and (especially) when the diet is completed and you are adjusting your daily intake to attain weight stabilization.

The problem of an "ideal" number of calories is compounded by many factors: age versus youth, for one (we do seem to require less to eat as we grow older *despite* activity); wide swings in day-to-day-activity (a woman who completes the greater part of her housework early in the week will naturally require more calories then; a man who sits behind a desk Monday through Friday and spends his weekends golfing or skiing just will not find an "exact" number of calories to consume on a *daily* basis); and—in the case of women—pregnancies and menstrual cycles.

It is suggested therefore that you stick as closely as possible to the Diet Ideal during the first three weeks, only adjusting it if your weight loss seems too slow or (remembering to keep initial fluid loss in mind) too rapid.

If you are convinced an adjustment is in order at that point—go ahead and make it, but continue to keep an eye on the scale, prepared to make another adjustment *after a suitable period*—say, two or three more weeks.

Attempting to adjust your eating day intake any more frequently than at two week intervals—whether the adjustment is upward or downward—*may* tend to compromise the habit factor. If you're losing at the rate of at least a pound-and-a-half a week—and yet your loss is not *so great* weekly that you feel continually tired (which, by the way, has not yet been known to happen to those who have pursued this diet)—I strongly urge you not to tamper with the Diet Ideal throughout the course of your weight loss, adjusting it only to achieve weight stability (if such an adjustment is necessary) when the diet has formally ended.

What about exercise, by the way? Do you recommend it in conjunction with this diet?

By all means—yes—*if* you are seeking to follow a program of exercise that you can continue with when the diet is completed (and if, of course, the exercise you choose is not overly severe for your present physical state; your doctor will know).

In the past, regular exercise has *not* been advised while dieting simply because people have tended to regard it as a *substitute* for dieting (which it is not) and some have complained it only makes them more hungry than ever—leading them to eat more than they should.

Today, however, most nutritionists *do* find sensible exercise advisable while dieting in that it helps tone the muscles, introduces large quantities of oxygen into the system, strengthens the heart and in general makes one *feel* healthier and more alert.

In addition, exercise *can help* reduce you!

A slow half-hour's walk on your eating day will burn up about 100 calories. If you walk moderately fast, you can burn 150 calories. A *very* fast half-hour's walk (at five miles per hour) will burn 325 calories!

If you're interested in jogging—and it is, in a way, a "natural" to tie in with your eating day—you can burn about 200 calories in a half-hour's jog (far less, you'll note, than walking *very* fast—and also far easier to maintain).

Various types of "light exercise" will burn up about 85 calories in half an hour.

However, I again caution you that because of the particular principle of the Eating Man's Diet, you should choose as an exercise one which you would like to maintain when the diet is ended. Even 15 minutes of light exercise daily will combust the equivalent of a full day's meals in two months. If you exercise *now*—and quit after the diet—the post-diet period of weight stabilization will be that much more difficult.

So if *your choice* is to exercise while on the diet, pick your method with the habit principle in mind . . . and then *wait out the diet's initial three-week period before assuming this new activity.*

Attempting to solve two problems at the same time—even such closely related ones—can lead to the solution of neither.

Speaking of problems, I've been intending to quit smoking for some time. Is there anything wrong with stopping on the day I begin the diet?

I can be much more definite about this answer.

Yes. There's quite a bit wrong with it.

Quit smoking *now*—or wait until the diet is completed.

Don't let a feeling of burgeoning strength delude you into taking on two tigers at the same time.

13

Other Considerations

Most diets seem to recommend daily weighings. I find though that the losses are so minute from day to day that they seem to frustrate more than help me. Might I weigh myself weekly with the Eating Man's Diet?

If you do not choose to weigh yourself on a daily basis, just be certain you decide on an interval of *even days* (such as the Saturday of one week followed by the Sunday of the next followed by the Saturday of the next, etc.) rather than *odd*—as you would on a true weekly basis.

As pointed out previously, the daily "swing" in weight from eating day to diet day may be as much as three pounds . . . and, on some occasions, more. Therefore you'll have a much closer idea of your *real* weight if you'll weigh yourself following an eating day.

However, as in other diets, it *is* recommended you weigh yourself on a daily basis—stripped—*at the same time of day* (preferably immediately after use of the bathroom facilities in the morning). In addition, the employment of a weight chart (such as found in the appendix) can pay big dividends by helping you *visualize* both your goal and your progress.

You will not feel as frustrated with daily weighings on the Eating Man's Diet as you may have with others simply because its "plateau" periods—when you feel as if you're never going to lose another pound—are neither as long-lasting nor as obvious.

On another diet you might seem to be "stuck" at a certain weight for as long as two or three weeks and then "rapidly lose" four or five pounds. When you weigh yourself daily under such conditions it's easy to see why you wonder if it's worth the time and effort. However, on the Eating Man's Diet you'll find that in addition to the comparatively wide day-to-day swing in poundage, losses tend to be almost immediately reflected after each eating day. Thus instead of the scale reading 175 for 14 days and then dropping to 170, your weight will be 175, then 172, then 174½, then 171½, etc. Keeping a daily chart under *these* conditions becomes more a pleasure than a task. And once you've kept your chart a month or so, your spirits—and your determination— will be buoyed each morning upon looking at it.

I have a weekly get-together with the girls on Wednesdays. In order to insure my being able to eat that night, might I put two diet days together—say Monday and Tuesday of each week?

Regular weekly get-togethers—whether they be for bowling, poker, bridge or just plain luncheons—make it impossible to both follow the Eating Man's Diet *and* enjoy "normal eating" on the day of the get-together.

You may *not* re-schedule your eating and diet days at such close interval and still hope to develop the habit principle of the diet. The every-other-day method becomes amazingly simple to follow only when it is conscientiously practiced on a consistent every-other-day basis. For this reason it is a great mistake to decide you're going to, for instance, diet every Monday, Wednesday, Friday and Sunday and *not* diet Tuesday, Thursday and Saturday. Stick with the every-other-day formula, continually exposing yourself to either eating or dieting on each and every day of the week and under all conceivable circumstances.

If you have to give up your bridge club every-other-week because the canapè temptations are just too great, rejoice in that you don't have to give it up *every* week—as you might find yourself having to do on a different type of diet.

Your best bet, of course, is to *not* give it up, *but not to break your diet either on that day.* Enjoy black coffee or tea with lemon while the other girls freely help themselves to the olives and anchovies. Holding off on that one day makes what you're missing that much more desirable—and enjoyable—when you're at last able to partake with a clear conscience. And such an exercise in sacrifice serves to remind you that by *continuing* to stick with the diet you'll one day be able to partake *every* week with a clear conscience—and a trim figure as well!

How often then MAY I adjust my eating and dieting days?

If possible, do not adjust them at all. Certainly an adjustment is out of the question during the first three crucial weeks.

If you wish to begin this diet as soon as possible, first sit down with a calendar and decide what events are coming up in the foreseeable future that you would prefer to have an eating day coincide with. Having made this determination, you can then arrange to begin the diet tomorrow—or on the following day.

In any case, *begin with a diet day rather than an eating day.*

The immediate feeling of weight loss—and it *will* be reflected on your scale the following morning—starts you off with considerable impetus while simplifying the task of arranging your first eating day meals—so that you can easily consume a good-sized breakfast and a good-sized lunch as well, both of which you will most certainly be looking forward to at the end of your first diet day.

Now should you find it advisable to make an occasional change in your diet/eating day schedule, do not make such a change more often than once a month and—to keep yourself honest—do it by putting two diet days together on the *first* such change and by putting two *eating* days together should there be a *second*.

Remember, I made only one such change in six months of dieting—and that was only in the very last month when I knew the habit couldn't be pried away from me with a crowbar.

Your choice is, quite simply, to *decide now* that you are going to stick with the every-other-day principle of the diet even if it does put a crimp in your social life *once in a while* or go with a diet that may put a *constant crimp* in it—with, most probably, no successful results—or, of course, remain overweight.

You suggest black coffee or tea with lemon on the diet day. Certainly we'd be allowed other low calorie choices.

Certainly is right.

The diet day listings in the appen
you a good idea of the wide scope
available (some highly nutritious, othe.
—not nutritious at all but, in their o
satisfying).

Here, in addition, is a selection of food
consume *almost at will* on your diet day wi.
your overdoing it (although I would ask you,
piece of mind, to note calorie content in the app
vegetables listed are low calorie *only* when eate.   or
with spices; they can become quite high in calo... ..s when
taken with butter or most salad dressings:

Asparagus	Lettuce
Bamboo shoots	Mushrooms
Bean sprouts	Mustard
Beet greens	Mustard greens
Beets	Okra
Bouillon	Paprika
Broccoli	Parsley
Brussels sprouts	Pepper (black, red and
Cabbage	green)
Carrots	Pimientos
Cauliflower	Radishes
Celery	Salt
Chard	Sauerkraut
Chewing gum (sugarless or	Scallions
not)	Soda water (seltzer)
Coffee (black)	Spices (all varieties)
Consomme	Spinach
Cucumbers	Squash, Butternut and
Dill pickles	Summer
Eggplant	String Beans
Endive	Tea (plain or with lemon)
Escarole	Tomatoes
Herbs (all varieties)	Turnips
Horseradish	Vinegar
Kale	Water
Leeks	Watercress

Not included on this list are a host of commercial diet
foods—such as artificial sweeteners (both saccharine and

clamate), low calorie carbonated beverages employ these sweeteners), and certain types of dietic candy and salad dressing—*which you may also use within reasonable limits,* having checked (in the case of the candy and the salad dressing) on the individual labels to determine exactly what the calorie content is.

Other commercial dietetic preparations may also be of interest to you. These include liquid and solid meals, every calorie of which is counted for you and appears on the product's label. Use them or not on the diet day—according to your own preference.

How about the use of these low calorie foods on the eating day? Do you recommend them then?

Yes—provided, of course, that you wish to make their use habitual—I very much recommend them.

An advantage of employing these low calorie foods as a substitute for high calorie foods is that you *may* learn you enjoy them just as much while benefitting dramatically in your daily calorie consumption.

For instance, if you now drink six cups of coffee daily with cream and sugar *and can learn* to enjoy it just as much black with an artificial sweetener, you may save as many as 600 calories a day right there! (Two *rounded* teaspoons of sugar = 70 calories. One tablespoon of real cream = 33.)

If you like to put three tablespoons of French dressing on your lettuce and tomatoes—and switch to a dietetic substitute—you can save as may as 265 calories per salad!

You can save 70 calories per highball by using low calorie gingerale instead of the regular.

I doubt very much, however, that you'll wish to consume a low calorie liquid lunch on a regular basis when your diet has ended; therefore it is not wise to have this *on your eating day* during the diet.

In any case, make certain that you *use* the calories you *save.* Do not congratulate yourself if you become so adept with low calorie substitutes that you find your calorie intake falling below the minimum required on that day. If you save 265 calories on your salad, make sure those 265 calories appear somewhere else in the meal!

As a bachelor I eat what I suppose is a disproportionately large number of complete frozen meals. Isn't there some

easy way of keeping track of their calorie content wi
having to add up the meat, the potatoes, the gravy, etc.?

Yes. Banquet Canning Company, Campbell Soup Company (maker of Swanson "TV" Dinners) and R. J. Reynolds
Foods, Inc. (who make Chun King Products) have been
kind enough to provide me with a complete calorie list of
their frozen dinners. Since these meals are uniform, con-
venient and often nutritionally complete, a selection of them
will be found in its own special section of the appendix's
calorie counter.

Would you clarify one point for me? When you speak of
the eating DAY and the diet DAY—do you consider it as a
true 24 hours (midnight to midnight) or as lasting from
sleep to sleep?

Sleep to sleep—sorry. Attempting to separate your "normal eating" from your dieting on a strictly time basis—as
you would with the separation point being midnight—can
lead too easily to your dieting all day, watching the *Tonight
Show* until midnight, and then really chowing down. It's
dangerous even if binge eating has never been a particular
problem of yours in the past—as it may well lead to it.

Separate the two days according to *natural cycles*—which
means considering that one ends and the other begins somewhere in the middle of your sleep.

Going to bed a little hungry after a diet day will help you
rise eagerly in the morning and head for that big breakfast.
And, as you'll find, there are few habits more satisfying to
establish than that of a truly hearty breakfast—which last
night's slightly empty feeling will help you enjoy.

My little boy is so heavy that he's very poor in sports and
is subject to the constant gibes of his friends. Would you
recommend the Eating Man's Diet for him?

It's especially important that you check with your doctor
before putting a child on *any* diet. Certainly an extremely
overweight child can benefit greatly from removing his excess
poundage—not only physically but emotionally as well.
Adults can tend to find other compensations for their weight
problems, whereas obese children see all that fat as a lead
weight about their self-esteem.

With your doctor's permission—and his help in deter-
mining both ideal weight and the on-off calorie consumption

vill undoubtedly find the Eating Man's Diet
any other you might help put him on. For one
gth of an unbroken regular diet—even if it's
veeks—can seem an eternity to a child. For
lren are much less inclined to let the word go
're dieting than adults are. (Their friends *can*
el.) As he follows the Eating Man's Diet his
see him eat ice cream and candy with them so
often that they just won't be aware of his pattern of *not*
eating them. And in the meantime, you'll be the instrument
of his forming lifetime sensible eating habits *early*.

*One last question. Aside from the psychological aspect of
the on-off pattern, can you suggest some other psychological
hints that might be applied to daily eating habits?*

Yes—as long as you understand that these are certainly
not original with *me*. But they are tested and true, and work
especially well in conjunction with the Eating Man's Diet in
that alone among diets, it allows you to begin practicing
these precepts immediately—rather than having to wait
several months until (if you're very lucky) you've shown a
substantial weight loss.

The three most useful—and easily practiced—psychological ploys that I found myself using on the diet (and still
use to some extent now) are:

1. Predetermining the meal.
2. Taking a break.
3. Leaving a little.

To predetermine your meal, all you need do is decide
beforehand exactly how much you will eat—including
everything from appetizer to dessert—and stick with that
determination!

I enjoy variety in food, and when I sit down to the dinner
table I find a salad and a bowl of soup before me along with,
most usually, a plate of appetizers: carrots, scallions, rad-
ishes, a couple of plum tomatoes, perhaps—and maybe a
little pickled herring. Before I start on these, however, I
generally pre-fill my plate from the main course: meat loaf,
a baked potato, peas, for instance—and then I help myself
to a piece of bread, carefully butter it and set it down at the
edge of my plate.

That picture (if you can visualize it) is worth a thousand desserts. (I generally *don't* have dessert with my supper meal, preferring to have it with lunch.) There, spread before me, is a variety of food that a nineteenth century king would have envied: Meat, soup, fish, bread, butter, and six varieties of vegetables—not counting the salad!

It's quite a *spread* all right—and since I've *predetermined* that this is *all* I'm going to eat, I can nibble at one thing and then at another, taking a considerable time before making any appreciable "dent" in any *one* of the various foods— thus almost inadvertently following another old stand-by: that of eating and chewing slowly. I *know* I'm not going to have *seconds*—a regular supper habit with me before I began this diet—so, realizing I'm restricted to only what I see before me, I may as well take my time and enjoy it. And so I do—both!

To take a break, (a habit I picked up from my wife who, as mother, cook and waitress for seven small children, nec- essarily has her supper interrupted any number of times), all you have to do is latch onto some excuse—good or bad— to get away from the table for just a minute or two.

You may—as I do—help feed the baby on occasion. Or you may suddenly decide this is the optimum time to check over your second grader's homework. Or maybe you can't stand the dog's whimpering any longer and decide it's time to fill up his plate or let him out in the yard. Running into the livingroom briefly to check the exact time and station of that TV show you plan to watch tonight is another fine excuse.

In any event, purposely turning your back on your food midway or two-thirds through the meal may make you sud- denly, surprisedly aware (as I continue to be) that you don't really need all that food as much as you thought you did. It's easy to develop a fascination with certain acts which propels you to continue performing them almost as a robot— yes, in a trance as it were—unless you have a sudden break along the way, which serves to make you aware of the rest of the world once more (including goals and plans of your own), thereby bringing you back to your "senses." Anyone who's watched TV—worked overtime—washed woodwork —or stayed out on the putting green—*far longer than he planned* is aware of this fascination syndrome. A planned break at the right time, however, can help you to hold any of these activities within reasonable limits. The same, of course, goes for eating.

In addition, when you return to the table with your break taken and see all that food still remaining, still waiting for you, the necessity of having to "begin again" makes you feel almost as if you're having two meals rather than one.

Leaving a little is probably the most difficult—and useful —of the three.

The corollary between obesity and cleaning one's plate (just as mother used to insist) is extremely high. The psychological reasons for this corollary are entirely too many to discuss in detail here.

However, let it suffice to say that you should always leave *something* behind—whether it's as little as a small crust of bread, a few peas, a scrap of lettuce *or* a sip of milk in your glass.

(If you've moral scruples against this practice—as many of the obese seemingly have—you must begin to persuade yourself that *you* are far more worth saving than an extra bite of bread. According to Dr. Louis Orr, past president of the American Medical Association, obesity is our *number one* health problem. It exceeds cancer, smoking, automobile accidents and whatever other dreaded disease or precondition for lasting bodily harm you may wish to name. Feed the scraps to the dog or the dispose-all. Don't make a dispose-all of yourself.)

The psychology of leaving a little something behind, of course, is that *you* are finished before the *food* is.

With the line being drawn by *you,* it's far easier to refuse to have any additional food. You're demonstrating in effect —even though it may not be true *at first*—that you've taken on all you can comfortably handle, and therefore all that food in the serving dishes and the refrigerator is certainly beyond your considering.

A most surprising psychological phenomenon is that *you* tend to react to your own actions in much the same way an *observer* would. In other words, your host—seeing you leave some food behind—will conclude: "I guess he's not hungry anymore." As strange as it seems, *you* tend to conclude the same thing about *yourself!*

Leave a little. There *will* be more to eat at your next meal.

14

The Pause Before the Plunge: Are You Ready?

It's squarely up to you now.

As you've studied the text of this book (or even checked out some of the appendix's charts and menus) a decision has slowly been forming within you. Perhaps you made up your mind early that you would follow the precepts of this diet—or perhaps your decision is all but complete. It *sounds* good to you—it's worth, you believe, giving it an honest try—and you've only to make the final commitment, nod your head, say yes . . . and psychologically put your signature to your new resolution's bottom line.

Now *if* you feel—what the heck—you'll look at your ideal weight and your ideal calorie consumption, you'll make a stab at a diet day tomorrow, in fact you'll give it a *couple* of days and see how it works out—please, don't even start.

For the chances of its working for you under these conditions, of doing what you want it to do, of bringing you down to your ideal weight (and then keeping you there) are very slim indeed.

In order to succeed at the Eating Man's Diet, you *must* have the real desire to lose weight. You *must* be determined that you've been a fatty, an overweight, an obesity long enough. *You must, in short, make the judgment that you are going to give the Eating Man's Diet not "a couple of days" but the full three habit-inducing weeks it calls for!*

"A couple of days" means nothing. Such a short-term "trial period" will help you no more and no less than the same length of time applied to any other diet. Remember, as was pointed out earlier in the book and as you no doubt fully realize from the many, many successes—seemingly inconsequential or not—that you have had throughout your life, a real resolve or determination—even though it may *seem* unsteady—is "the necessary big first step" in *any* program . . . and most certainly in this one.

You *won't* find those first three weeks so "easy" that they seem to happen automatically for you.

You *must* approach them (if you are to succeed) with all the determination, vigor and cunning that you approach the beginning of any new, worthwhile (and initially difficult) habit.

Don't—because, admittedly, it *can* look easy—make the mistake of approaching the diet half-heartedly, without adequate preparation.

All right, fine, you say. *How do I prepare?*

First—although I'm sure that by now you've grown tired of hearing me say this—check with your doctor. Get his stamp of approval. Such a step is important not only as a commonsense health measure, but also because once you've done it, you've cleared the final *outside obstacle* out of the way. With his saying yes, any other obstacles are necessarily *internal*—and you're quite capable of handling them yourself.

Next (and please bear in mind, I'm urging this upon you only on the assumption that you do question your determination; if you *know* you're ready, skip this and start now!) further prepare yourself mentally by considering every *negative* reason you may have for losing weight.

Look at yourself in the mirror. Go ahead. Strip completely. Stand in front of a full-length mirror and *stare*. Get front, side and even back views. Let yourself—if you dare—jiggle up and down a little (or are you too concerned about what a devastating effect *that* will have?). Slip on trunks or a bikini and let your mate snap your picture. There are a host of places—some nationally advertised—that will be happy to blow your snapshots into poster-sized portraits for three to five dollars. Decorate the wall of one of your private rooms with them. Put them somewhere *you* will see them frequently—but friends dropping in will not. (Mine—both *before* and, thankfully, *after* posters—stare at me from the walls of my den as I write this.) Your first three weeks will probably have elapsed by the time the shots have been processed and returned from the poster company.

In addition, *think hard* about the very real problems of being overweight (not only the obvious medical ones; unless your excessive weight has actually caused you illness it's hard not to think: "Well, *I'll* be the lucky one—*my* heart won't fail early!"). But think about the real difficulties it has already aroused—and if you've been fat for any length of time, they are many.

Consider the sports you never excelled in, the tears that flowed so freely when you didn't get to go to that dance. Think about your husband: He tells you he loves you just as you are—and God bless him for that. But like any other husband he's human. *Day after day there are girls at the office* . . . so went a popular song of a few years back. Even if he would never be untrue—is it *easy* for him? Or *hard?*

Think of your wife. Oh sure, there's nobody else in the world for her but you. And "as everybody knows," obesity doesn't make nearly the difference in a man that it does in a woman. But *she* knows obesity can also be far more dangerous in a man—and if you won't worry about it, she will. Male or female, the chances of dropping dead from a "heart attack" are twice as great if you're as little as 20 per cent over your ideal weight. The only thing is, *if you're a man you'll probably have this attack 20 years sooner.* Is it worth it to worry her with such unwelcome statistics? Will your insurance really fill the gap in her life—and in the lives of your children? Besides, how long do you think she'll tolerate your letting yourself go to pot (literally!) before she decides against the bother of keeping *herself* trim? (You've noticed, I'm sure, that obesity can spread like any other disease in a family.)

From the exertion of polishing your shoes to the worry over what sort of an impression you'll make on the new boss or client, there are scores of reasons—negative ones— why it would pay you to reduce.

Get a piece of paper. *Write down five of them.* The ones you consider most important. (I'd leave space for them here, but you may be reluctant—as are most people—to put personal notes where they might fall into another's hands.) Keep this piece of paper where you can look at it frequently. And *do* look at it.

And, while you're at it, put down some *positive* reasons as well. Three will do—as those which are strictly positive are generally more difficult to come by.

How about estimating how long the diet will take—and making those three reasons some very enjoyable undertakings you'd like to pursue upon its conclusion?

Will your husband buy you a complete new wardrobe if you get your figure down to its ideal size? (He *might,* you know. You can *ask* him.)

Indeed, will the ending of your diet coincide with July at the beach? Or with the Christmas family reunion you've long hoped to help arrange? Can your vacation be scheduled (with appropriate leeway) so that you can enjoy the shows in New York, the mountains of Colorado or the rides at Disneyland as a reward for a job well done?

Engaged to be married? What nicer present than a *permanently slim you* can you bestow upon your new spouse?

Think. You'll come up with three good *positive* reasons.

And then consider—*before* you start—just what sort of difficulties the first three weeks will entail and how you can best handle them. Does your mate tend to kid you when you take on a diet? ("Oh no—not another one!") What's your best approach to putting up with the wisecracks—besides the incontrovertible evidence you'll soon have that 1) you are actually losing weight this time; 2) he's not permanently deprived of your companionable enjoyment of mealtimes—whether you happen to be dining *in* or *out* (the "social enjoyment of food" is one of the most important aspects of eating—and one of other diets' greatest stumbling blocks); and 3) for the first time—including even the diet you undertook with the aid of tranquilizers—your nerves are not on the verge of being shattered with each pound you lose.*

* Verplanck points out truly that "people on crash diets often become intolerably bad-tempered, and have to watch their relationships with other people. The (Eating Man's Diet) minimizes this probability."

What are you going to do when it gets *rough?* (And believe me, it most probably *will* at one time or another in those first three weeks.) What about the morning that—for no good reason, as we all say—you wake up depressed, in a blue funk, feeling sorry for yourself? And, as luck would have it, here it is a diet day! Only 900 calories allowed. Do you think you can hang on, persevere, get through that *one day* somehow?

Or how about on the eating day when you've finished your quota of food and *full well realize* that it's quite a bit more than possible for you to *continue* eating—to have just a little extra? When your tendency is to eat compulsively —as I, one who long had the habit, certainly know—the fact that you *can* eat more leads easily to the thought that you *must* eat more. This may be the hardest moment of the diet for you. (It was for me.) Can you—not through habit, not through design, but perhaps only through sheer grit—resist this almost overpowering temptation and hold off *for only the first three weeks?*

If you can give thoughtful, positive answers to these last several questions you are more than ready to begin your own customized version of the Eating Man's Diet.

I should point out, however, that the situation over the first three weeks needn't be nearly as bleak as I may have depicted it. Some *have* found the first three weeks amazingly easy—and in fact encountered *no* great problems from start to finish. I *hope* this is you.

Others have run into one problem or another—and handled them with far more ease than they would have imagined.

But I've emphasized them here for the simple reason that I do not wish to lead you to believe the diet is one bit easier than it actually is. If you enter upon it with great enthusiasm, half in love with the whole idea before you start, and it works out quite the way you thought and hoped it would—well, fine. If, on the other hand, you begin it with the same spirit—and encounter *unexpected* pitfalls along the way—you're likely to be discouraged and make the mistake of thinking it will not work for you.

There *are* pitfalls. You may leap grandly over them, walk

cautiously around them, or even stumble into one or two. I just wish to make certain you know they are there.

Look forward to the end of those first three weeks! Once they've passed . . . once the diet's habit principle has begun to take root . . . you will *still* have to bring some effort to your program each day, but it will be the effort of keeping an already rolling ball rolling—not the effort of starting it anew every time you sit down to a meal.

This habit which you await—and which you can confidently expect—does *not* imply that you'll tumble out of bed one morning 21 days from now feeling like an entirely new person. (Did you feel like a new person on the day you knew you'd licked the habit of biting your nails, cracking your knuckles, arriving late for work or standing in a slumped position?) What it *does* mean is that as you apply effort to your diet regimen yourself, you'll feel an unexpected aid—an assist, if you like—making your effort that much easier.

It's as if you daily practiced lifting weights. At first 50 pounds might be very, very hard to put over your head. After some weeks of effort, however, habit (as embodied in newly developed muscle power) will make putting that weight over your head quite simple. *As small as the effort is, it still remains an effort, however—and in order to get that weight up there YOU will have to make that effort.*

But take heart. You are about to enter upon a program that for the first time, perhaps, will find you *satisfied* with (relatively) little food rather than *unsatisfied* with (relatively) a lot.

And it'll go fast for you.

As you may have already figured, a Diet Ideal of as much as 2000 calories alternating with 900 will bring your diet to an end even faster than that of a steady 1500 day after day.

A Diet Ideal of 2300 calories will take only *seven per cent longer.*

Even a Diet Ideal of 3000 calories will take only *30 per cent (!)* longer than a straight 1500 schedule.

And in each of these cases, with the constant breaks, the Eating Man's Diet will *seem* so much faster—and you have so much more to benefit by it, both in the sureness of your completing it—and in the ease of maintaining your new weight level once the job is done.

So—when do you start?

Before you close the covers of this book, make that decision.

It *can* be tomorrow . . . it *can* be the next day . . . it *must* be sometime this week! Don't make the mistake of waiting until after New Year's—or your next birthday.

Pick any one of the upcoming seven days as your personal D-day. If you feel you *want* to do it—if you feel *ready* to go—pick that day right now. Put it off longer than a week and chances are you'll *never* get at it.

You decide. It's *entirely* up to you.

But for your own sake—*decide now!*

"To be fat, to be hated," wrote William Shakespeare in *Henry IV, Part I.* True—and no one hates a fat man more than he himself does. This is your opportunity to turn that self-hate into the self-love and self-respect you may have long denied yourself—and which you'll find you most certainly deserve.

"Imprisoned in every fat man," said Cyril Connolly in *The Unquiet Grave,* "a thin one is wildly signaling to be let out."

Let him out. (And let *her* out.)

It's time, don't you think?

Eating Man's Diet
Appendix

CHART A—YOUR IDEAL WEIGHT
CHART B—RECOMMENDED CALORIE CONSUMPTION
CHART C—YOUR DAILY WEIGHT RECORD
COMPARISON CALORIE COUNTER (With Special
    Frozen Dinner Section)
A GUIDE TO YOUR DAILY NUTRITIONAL "MUSTS"
EATING MAN'S DIET MENUS (From 600 to 3500
    Calories Per Day)

YOUR IDEAL WEIGHT

The following tables—for both men and women—are estimations of *desirable* weight: what your bathroom scale should read in the morning as you mount it *without clothes*. The heights given are, of course, how tall you stand *shoeless*.

MEN—25 AND OVER

Height		Small Frame	Medium Frame	Large Frame
5	1	107–115	113–124	121–136
5	2	110–118	116–128	124–139
5	3	113–121	119–131	127–143
5	4	116–124	122–134	130–147
5	5	119–128	125–138	133–151
5	6	123–132	129–142	137–156
5	7	127–136	133–147	142–161
5	8	131–140	137–151	146–165
5	9	135–145	141–155	150–169
5	10	139–149	145–160	154–174
5	11	143–153	149–165	159–179
6	0	147–157	153–170	163–184
6	1	151–162	157–175	168–189
6	2	155–166	162–180	173–194
6	3	159–170	167–185	177–199

WOMEN—25 AND OVER

Height		Small Frame	Medium Frame	Large Frame
4	8	87– 93	91–102	99–114
4	9	89– 96	93–105	101–117
4	10	91– 99	96–108	104–120
4	11	94–102	99–111	107–123
5	0	97–105	102–114	110–126
5	1	100–108	105–117	113–129
5	2	103–111	108–121	116–133
5	3	106–114	111–125	120–137
5	4	109–118	115–130	124–141
5	5	113–122	119–134	128–145
5	6	117–126	123–138	132–149
5	7	121–130	127–142	136–153
5	8	125–135	131–146	140–158
5	9	129–139	135–150	144–163
5	10	133–143	139–154	148–168

RECOMMENDED CALORIE CONSUMPTION

Here are the listings—for both men and women—of recommended daily calorie consumption depending on ideal weight and usual activity. The Diet Ideal—the midpoint between the minimum and maximum rounded off by no more than 25 calories —is the number of calories one should consistently aim at on the "eating day" throughout the diet. With the diet completed, one should continue to consume *approximately* this number on a daily basis—adjusting it upward or downward in order to maintain a stabilized weight. (See Chapter 11: *Your Own Diet —Custom-Made.*)

Ideal Weight	DAILY CALORIE ALLOWANCE Minimum	*Diet Ideal*	Maximum
90	1350	*1600*	1800
95	1425	*1650*	1900
100	1500	*1750*	2000
105	1575	*1850*	2100
110	1650	*1900*	2200
115	1725	*2000*	2300
120	1800	*2100*	2400
125	1875	*2200*	2500
130	1950	*2300*	2600
135	2025	*2350*	2700
140	2100	*2450*	2800
145	2175	*2550*	2900
150	2250	*2600*	3000

Ideal Weight	DAILY CALORIE ALLOWANCE Minimum	*Diet Ideal*	Maximum
155	2325	*2700*	3100
160	2400	*2800*	3200
165	2475	*2900*	3300
170	2550	*3000*	3400
175	2625	*3050*	3500
180	2700	*3150*	3600
185	2775	*3250*	3700
190	2850	*3300*	3800
195	2925	*3400*	3900
200	3000	*3500*	4000

On the last page of this book you will find a lined—but otherwise blank—chart. This is your daily weight record and it will easily see you through the first two months of the program.

For you to do: Using a razor blade or scissors, carefully detach this page from the rest of the book.

Fill in your name (your first name will do); your present weight; your ideal weight; your minimum, Diet Ideal and maximum calorie allowances; and the date of your beginning the Eating Man's Diet *(sometime this week, remember).* You may *pencil in* the date you hope to complete the diet—based on the realistic calculation of 1½ to 2½ pounds per week—or leave it blank (and fill it in later!).

If you have no more than 20 pounds to lose, enter your present weight in the left-hand margin opposite the graph's top line, your present weight *minus two* opposite the line directly beneath, and so on down to the bottom line. (For instance: 140, 138, 136, 134, etc.)

If you must lose between 20 and 50 pounds, also work your way down from your present weight in the left-hand margin—but in units of five. (For instance: 180, 175, 170, 165, etc.)

Over 50 pounds to lose, again descend from your present weight—but in units of 10. (220, 210, 200, 190, etc.)

With that taken care of, note that every *fifth* vertical line is somewhat longer than the others. Above each of these longer lines enter the appropriate date *at ten-day increments.* (Thus, if your diet begins on June 27, the dates running across the top of the graph will read: July 7, July 17, July 27, August 6, etc.)

Your weight chart is now *personalized*—quite as customized to your needs as the Eating Man's Diet itself is. Scotch-tape it inside the door of your medicine cabinet so that you'll be able to mark down your weight immediately after your morning's weigh-in.

Notate your weight not by dots but by a continuous jagged line with the level following each eating day being marked on a vertical line—the level after each diet day falling in the space *between* the lines.

You will now not only have a complete picture of your losses over the first two months—as divided into significant ten-day periods, but by "reading across" the vertical lines only, you'll be able to keep constant check on your "real" weight level: that which follows a full day of eating.

Should your diet take any longer than the space provided, simply use this chart to trace another one!

COMPARISON CALORIE COUNTER*
(With Special Frozen Dinner Section)

Alcoholic Beverages
Beverages, Miscellaneous
Breads, Grains & Cereals
Dairy Products & Eggs
Dressings & Oils
Fish & Seafood
Fruits & Juices
Meat & Poultry
Sauces, Relishes, Sugar & Spices
   Sauces
   Relishes
   Sugar
   Spices
Soups & Broths
Sweets
   Candies, Nuts & T.V. Snacks
   Cakes, Pies & Cookies
   Miscellaneous Desserts & Sweets
Vegetables

SPECIAL FROZEN DINNER SECTION

ALCOHOLIC BEVERAGES

Item	Portion	Calories
Ale	1 glass (8 oz.)	100
Bacardi Rum	1½ oz.	100
Beer	1 glass (8 oz.)	100
Benedictine Cordial	1 oz.	75
Blackberry Brandy	1½ oz.	75
Blackberry Cordial	1 oz.	100
Bock Beer	1 glass (8 oz.)	175
Bordeaux Wine	1 wine glass	125
Bourbon	1½ oz.	100

* (Note: Never count your calories in a hurry. The Comparison Calorie Counter—which groups foods together according to type rather than running them in unvaried alphabetical order—is intentionally designed to allow you to make comparisons between similar foods even as you look up your daily menu. Thus you may discover you'd rather have two servings of potatoes mashed with milk and butter than one serving of french fries—at a saving of 150 calories. You might prefer three glasses of regular beer over two glasses of bock—at a saving of 50 calories, etc.)

Bourbon highball	1 glass (8 oz.)	150
Brandy	1½ oz.	100
Brandy Alexander	1 cocktail glass	240
Brandy, Apricot	1 glass	75
Brandy Egg Nog	1 cup	300
Brandy Punch	1 cup	225
Bronx Cocktail	1 cocktail glass	225
Burgundy Wine	1 wine glass	85
Chablis	1 wine glass	75
Champagne	1 cocktail	100
Chartreuse Cordial	1 oz.	75
Claret Wine	1 wine glass	75
Cognac	1½ oz.	75
Cordial	1 cordial glass	80
Creme de Cocoa	1 oz.	75
Creme de Menthe	1 oz.	75
Cuba Libre	1 cocktail glass	225
Daiquiri	1 cocktail glass	125
French Vermouth (Dry)	2 oz.	35
Gin Alexander	1 cocktail glass	225
Gin Buck	6 oz.	150
Gin Collins	1 glass	150
Gin Fizz	1 glass	125
Gin Rickey	1 glass	150
Gin & Tonic	1 glass	125
Half & Half (Beer & Stout)	1 glass (8 oz.)	125
Highball	1 average	150
Hot Grog	6 oz.	175
Hot Toddy	1 cup	150
Irish Whiskey	1½ oz.	100
Italian Vermouth	2 oz.	50
Lime Rickey	1 glass	175
Madeira Wine	1 wine glass	75
Martini	1 cocktail glass	125
Mint Julep	1 glass	215
Old Fashioned	1 cocktail glass	150
Old Fashioned (Scotch)	1 cocktail glass	175
Peach Brandy	1½ oz.	75
Pink Lady	1 cocktail glass	175
Rhine Wine	1 wine glass	75
Rock Rye	1 cocktail glass	225
Rum Carioca	1 glass	100
Rum & Cola	1 glass	175
Rum Cooler	1 glass	225
Rum Egg Nog	1 glass	300

Rum, Hot Buttered	1 cup	150
Rye Whiskey	1½ oz.	100
Sauterne (Dry)	1 wine glass	75
Sauterne (Sweet)	1 wine glass	100
Scotch Whiskey	1½ oz.	100
Scotch & Soda	1 glass	100
Sherry Wine	1 wine glass	125
Sloe Gin	1 oz.	75
Sloe Gin Fizz	1 glass	150
Sparkling Burgundy	1 wine glass	90
Tokay Wine	1 wine glass	70
Tom Collins	1 glass	175
Tom & Jerry	1 glass	175
Vermouth	1½ oz.	50
Vodka	1 oz.	125
Whiskey Sour	1 cocktail glass	125
White Wine	1 wine glass	135

BEVERAGES, MISCELLANEOUS

Carbonated Beverages (Regular)	1 glass (6 oz.)	75
Carbonated Beverages (Low Cal.)	1 glass (6 oz.)	1 to 6
Coffee (Black)	—	0
Fruit Punch	1 glass (6 oz.)	150
Ginger Beer	1 glass (6 oz.)	75
Ice Cream Soda	1 average	350
Lemonade	1 glass (6 oz.)	100
Postum (Black)	1 cup	10
Soda Water (Seltzer)	—	0
Tea (Black)	—	0
Water	—	0

BREADS, GRAINS & CEREALS

All Bran Cereal	1 cup	140
Bagel	1	100
Barley	½ cup	325
Bisquick Flour	½ cup	365
Biscuits—		
Baking powder	1 large	100
Buttermilk	1 large	110
Short Cake	1 large	175
Tortoni	1 small	175
Yeast	1 large	100
Boston Brown Bread	1 slice	75

Boston Brown Muffin	1 average	110
Bran Bread	1 slice	75
Bran Flakes	¾ cup	100
Bran Muffins	1 average	100
Bread—		
Cracked Wheat	1 slice	60
Egg	1 slice	75
French	1 slice	60
Garlic	1 slice	85
Ginger	2″ square	175
Gluten	1 slice	75
Italian	1 slice	65
Protein	1 slice	50
Raisin	1 slice	85
Rye	1 slice	85
Vienna	1 slice	60
White	1 slice	75
Whole Wheat	1 slice	75
Buckwheat Flour	½ cup	240
Caraway Rolls	1 average	125
Cereal—		
Cooked	1 cup	150
Dry (Most—Unsweetened)	1 cup	110
Puffed Rice & Wheat	1 cup	65
Cinnamon Roll	1 average	100
Corn Bread	1 slice	200
Corn Meal	½ cup (cooked)	60
Corn Meal Flour	½ cup	240
Corn Muffin	1 average	100
Crackers—		
Graham	4	55
Oyster	1 cup	120
Round	1 average	15
Ry-Krisp	3	50
Saltine	2″ square	15
Soda	2½″ square	25
Whole Rye	1	20
Crepe Suzettes	1	225
Croutons	6 cubes	25
Dumpling	1	275
English Muffin	1 average	150
Flour	1 cup	400
French Rolls	1	100
French Toast	1	125
Hard Rolls	1	100

Hot Cross Buns	1	150
Kaiser Rolls	1	125
Macaroni	1 cup	200
Matzoh	1 average	125
Melba Toast	1	30
Milk Toast	1	170
Onion Roll	1	150
Pancakes	3 average	250
Parkerhouse Rolls	1	100
Plain Rolls	1 small	75
Popcorn	1 cup	50
Popovers	1	100
Pretzels—		
Stick	5 medium	20
Twist	6 average	100
Rice—		
Boiled (White)	¾ cup	100
Brown	¾ cup	100
Chinese Fried	1 cup	200
Flour	½ cup	350
Fried	1 cup	200
Mexican	1 cup	225
Spanish	1 cup	125
Wild (Cooked)	¾ cup	110
Steamed	½ cup	100
Roman Meal	½ cup	125
Waffle	1 average	225
Whole Wheat Muffin	1	125
Zwieback	1	30

DAIRY PRODUCTS & EGGS

Butter (or Margarine)	1 pat	50
Cheese—		
American	2 tbsp. (1 slice)	100
Bleu	2 tbsp.	100
Brick	2 tbsp.	100
Brie	2 tbsp.	85
Camembert	2 tbsp.	85
Cheddar	2 tbsp.	100
Cottage	1 cup	200
Creamed	2 tbsp.	100
Gorganzola	2 tbsp.	70
Gouda	2 tbsp.	85
Gruyere	2 tbsp.	100

Liederkranz	2 tbsp.	85
Limburger	2 tbsp.	100
Neufchatel	2 tbsp.	100
Parmesan	2 tbsp.	100
Provolone	2 tbsp.	70
Romano	2 tbsp.	120
Roquefort	2 tbsp.	70
Scamorze	1 oz.	100
Stilton	2 tbsp.	100
Swiss	2 tbsp. (1 slice)	100
Cream—		
Heavy	1 tbsp.	50
Light	1 tbsp.	33
Sour	¼ cup	200
Whipped	1 tbsp.	50
Eggs—		
Fried with Fat	1 large	115
Fried without Fat	1 large	80
Raw, Boiled, Baked	1 large	80
Raw White	Each	20
Raw Yolk	Each	60
Egg Nog	1 cup	300
Egg Roll	1 average	175
Ice Cream (All Flavors)	1 scoop	150
Milk—		
Buttermilk	1 cup	85
Chocolate	1 cup	225
Condensed	1 tbsp.	60
Evaporated (Sweet)	1 tbsp.	40
Evaporated (Unsweet)	½ cup	50
Goats'	1 cup	165
Malted	1 glass (8 oz.)	400
Shake	1 glass (8 oz.)	350
Skimmed	1 glass (8 oz.)	90
Whole	1 glass (8 oz.)	165
Yogurt (plain)	1 cup	150

DRESSINGS & OILS

Bacon Fat	1 tbsp.	50
Boiled Salad Dressing	¼ cup	100
Cooking Oil (Veg.)	1 tbsp.	100
Cottonseed Oil	1 tbsp.	100
Crisco	1 tbsp.	100
French Dressing	1 tbsp.	100

Garlic Dressing	1 tbsp.	100
Low Calorie Dressing (Most)	1 tbsp.	12
Mayonnaise	1 tbsp.	100
Mazola Oil	1 tbsp.	100
Mineral Oil	—	0
Olive Oil	1 tbsp.	125
Peanut Oil	1 tbsp.	100
Roquefort Dressing	1 tbsp.	125
Russian Dressing	1 tbsp.	50
Thousand Islands Dressing	1 tbsp.	100

FISH & SEAFOOD

Anchovy Paste	1 tbsp.	50
Barracuda	aver. svg.	135
Bass	¼ lb.	100
Bluefish, Baked	aver. svg.	200
Bluefish, Broiled	aver. svg.	185
Bluefish, Fried	aver. svg.	325
Buffalo Fish	aver. svg.	115
Butter Fish	aver. svg.	200
Carp	aver. svg.	100
Catfish	aver. svg.	100
Caviar	1 tbsp.	50
Clams	12 medium	100
Clams, Deviled	6 medium	100
Clams, Fried	6 medium	200
Codfish	aver. svg.	100
Codfish Balls	1 average	100
Codfish, Creamed	½ cup	150
Codfish, Dried	4 oz.	400
Crab	½ cup	65
Crab, Deviled	1 medium	200
Eel (Baked or Broiled)	aver. svg.	185
Flounder	aver. svg.	150
Frog Legs	4 large	50
Gefuelte Fish	aver. svg.	150
Haddock, Broiled	aver. svg.	180
Haddock, Creamed	aver. svg.	230
Haddock, Fried	aver. svg.	250
Hake	aver. svg.	125
Halibut, Broiled	aver. svg.	200
Halibut, Creamed	aver. svg.	250
Herring, Kippered	aver. svg.	225
Herring, Pickled	aver. svg.	150

Herring, Smoked	aver. svg.	225
Lobster—	aver. svg.	100
Cocktail	½ cup	90
Creamed	aver. svg.	150
Egg Foo Yung	aver. svg.	275
Newburg	aver. svg.	350
Lox	2 oz.	200
Mackerel	aver. svg.	175
Mussels	12	125
Oysters—		
Baked	12	85
Blue Point	12	100
Fried	6	250
On Half Shell	6	50
Raw	6	50
Rockefeller	6	180
Perch	aver. svg.	100
Pompano	aver. svg.	125
Porgy	aver. svg.	100
Red Snapper—		
Baked	aver. svg.	100
Broiled	aver. svg.	100
Creole	aver. svg.	150
Salmon—		
Baked	aver. svg.	250
Broiled	aver. svg.	225
Canned, Pink	aver. svg.	160
Canned, Red	aver. svg.	190
Loaf	aver. svg.	225
Nova Scotia	2 oz.	200
Sand Babs	aver. svg.	125
Sardines	4	100
Scallops	aver. svg.	400
Shad—		
Baked	aver. svg.	190
Broiled	aver. svg.	125
Shad Roe	aver. svg.	100
Shrimp—		
Boiled	10	100
Creole	aver. svg.	175
Egg Foo Yung	aver. svg.	275
French Fried	10	200
Fried	aver. svg.	250
Smelt	7	100
Sole (Broiled, Fillet)	aver. svg.	125

Squid	aver. svg.	125
Sturgeon	2 oz.	175
Swordfish	aver. svg.	150
Terrapin	aver. svg.	150
Trout	½ lb.	225
Tuna—		
Cooked	¾ cup	100
In Oil	¼ cup	125
Whitefish—		
Broiled	aver. svg.	125
Fried	aver. svg.	225
Smoked	aver. svg.	150
Steamed	aver. svg.	125

FRUITS & JUICES

Apple—		
Baked	1 large	200
Butter	1 tbsp.	35
Cider	1 cup	100
Juice	1 cup	125
Raw	1 medium	75
Sauce (w/Sugar)	1 cup	200
Apricot—		
Canned	3 halves	50
Dried	3	40
Juice	6 oz.	120
Raw	1	20
Banana	1	100
Blackberries		
Fresh	1 cup	100
Canned (w/Syrup)	1 cup	200
Canned (w/Water)	1 cup	100
Juice	6 oz.	75
Blueberries—		
Canned (w/Syrup)	½ cup	125
Canned (w/Water)	½ cup	50
Fresh	1 cup	100
Boysenberries	1 cup	100
Boysenberry Juice	6 oz.	75
Cantaloupe	½ medium	50
Casaba Melon	¼ average	120
Cherries—		
Fresh	½ cup	50
Maraschino	2 aver.	35

Coconut (Fresh)	1 slice (2″ x 1″)	100
Coconut Milk	1 cup	60
Cranberry Sauce	3 tbsp.	100
Dates	4	100
Figs—		
Canned	½ cup	125
Dried	1	50
Fresh	4 small	125
Fruit Cocktail	1 cup	200
Grapefruit—		
Canned	½ cup	75
Fresh	½ small	50
Juice (Sweetened)	3 oz.	45
Juice (Unsweetened)	3 oz.	30
Grapes—		
Fresh	1 cup	100
Juice	4 oz.	75
Honeydew Melon	¼ aver.	65
Huckleberries (Fresh)	½ cup	50
Kumquats—		
Candied	1	25
Fresh	6 medium	70
Lemons—		
Fresh	1 medium	30
Juice	½ cup	30
Loganberries—		
Canned	½ cup	45
Fresh	½ cup	45
Juice	6 oz.	80
Mango	1 aver.	120
Muskmelon	½ medium	50
Nectarines—		
Fresh	1 medium	70
Juice	6 oz.	100
Oranges—		
Fresh	1 medium	75
Juice (Fresh)	6 oz.	75
Juice (Canned, Swtnd)	4 oz.	70
Juice (Canned, Unswtnd)	4 oz.	55
Papaya	½ cup	35
Papaya Juice	6 oz.	75
Peach—		
Canned	2 halves	50
Fresh	1 medium	50

Pear—		
Canned	2 halves	75
Fresh	1 medium	75
Juice	4 oz.	55
Persimmon	1 medium	100
Pineapple—		
Canned	½ cup	200
Fresh	1 cup	75
Juice	1 cup	125
Plums—		
Canned	2 medium	75
Fresh	1	30
Pomegranate—		
Fresh	1	100
Juice	6 oz.	100
Prunes—		
Cooked	3	100
Dried	4	100
Juice	½ cup	85
Raisins	½ cup	225
Raspberries—		
Canned	½ cup	100
Fresh	½ cup	50
Juice	6 oz.	100
Rhubarb (Stewed w/Sugar)	½ cup	200
Strawberries—		
Canned or Frozen	1 cup	225
Fresh	1 cup	50
Tangerine—		
Fresh	1 large	35
Juice	½ cup	50
Watermelon—		
Fresh	1 medium slice	100
Pickled Rind	½ cup	40

MEAT & POULTRY

Bacon—		
Broiled	1 slice	40
Canadian	4 oz.	250
Beef—		
Barbecued	aver. svg.	300
Boiled	aver. svg.	250
Brains	6 oz.	200

Burgers	3 oz.	300
Chili Con Carne	½ cup	200
Chop Suey	½ cup	275
Chow Mein	½ cup	150
Corned	4 oz.	250
Curried	aver. svg.	400
Dried	3 oz.	175
Filet Mignon	aver. svg.	250
Hash	4 oz.	125
Heart	3 oz.	100
Liver	aver. svg.	150
Loaf	aver. svg.	225
Pot Pie	8 oz.	450
Roast	aver. svg.	200
Steak	aver. svg.	225
Stew	1 cup	250
Stroganoff	aver. svg.	350
Tongue	2 slices	100
Tripe	4 oz.	175
Bologna	1 medium slice	85
Chicken—		
A la King	½ cup	375
Baked	aver. svg.	200
Cacciatore	aver. svg.	225
Canned	4 oz.	225
Capon	aver. svg.	225
Chop Suey	½ cup	275
Chow Mein	½ cup	125
Curried	aver. svg.	325
Egg Foo Yung	aver. svg.	350
Fricassee	aver. svg.	225
Giblets	aver. svg.	150
Livers	each	50
Liver, Chopped	1 oz.	125
Pie	aver. svg.	500
Roasted ⁻	aver. svg.	200
Salad	aver. svg.	225
Stewed	½ medium	225
Chitterlings	aver. svg.	250
Duck, Roasted	aver. svg.	300
Goose, Roasted	aver. svg.	175
Guinea Hen	aver. svg.	175
Ham—	aver. slice	100
Deviled	1 tbsp.	100

Butt (Boiled)	aver. slice	100
Fried	2 slices	200
Hock	aver. svg.	450
Steak	aver. svg.	400
Lamb—		
Chop, Broiled	1 medium	200
Roast	aver. svg.	200
Stew	aver. svg.	250
Tongue	2 slices	100
Liverwurst	3″ x ¼″ slice	75
Mutton	aver. svg.	200
Oxtail	aver. svg.	250
Pheasant, Roast	aver. svg.	175
Pork—		
Barbecued Spare Ribs	6 ribs	250
Chop (Broiled or Baked)	1 medium	225
Chop Suey	½ cup	300
Chow Mein	½ cup	175
Egg Foo Yung	aver. svg.	475
Kidney	aver. svg.	130
Loin Roast	1 slice	100
Sweet & Sour	aver. svg.	250
Quail	aver. svg.	175
Rabbit	aver. svg.	175
Sausage—		
Frankfurter	2 medium	250
Knockwurst	1 medium	250
Pork Links	4 links	300
Salami	1 oz.	125
Vienna	4 oz.	300
Squab	½ medium	200
Turkey—		
Canned	4 oz.	300
Hash	aver. svg.	175
Roast	aver. svg.	175
Veal—		
Birds	2 aver.	350
Chop	1 medium	150
Cutlet (Broiled)	aver. svg.	125
Loaf	aver. svg.	250
Roast	aver. svg.	150
Scallopini	aver. svg.	375
Steak	aver. svg.	250
Stew	aver. svg.	250

SAUCES

A-1 Sauce	1 tsp.	10
Barbecue Sauce	1 tbsp.	50
Catsup	1 tbsp.	25
Chili Sauce	1 tbsp.	25
Cranberry Sauce	3 tbsp.	100
Cream Sauce	2 tbsp.	50
Fudge Sauce	1 tbsp.	50
Garlic Sauce	1 tbsp.	100
Gravy	1 tbsp.	50
Hard Sauce	1 tbsp.	100
Hollandaise Sauce	1 tbsp.	75
Lemon Sauce	1 tbsp.	25
Lobster Sauce	1 tbsp.	40
Maple Syrup	1 tbsp.	60
Mint Sauce	1 tbsp.	50
Mustard	1 tbsp.	10
Seafood Cocktail Sauce	1 tbsp.	50
Shish Kebab Sauce	1 tbsp.	25
Tartar Sauce	1 tbsp.	100
Tomato Sauce	¼ cup	50
White Sauce	1 tbsp.	25
Wine Sauce	1 tbsp.	35
Worcestershire Sauce	1 tbsp.	15

RELISHES

Horseradish	1 tbsp.	5
Olives	6 small	50
Picallili	1 tbsp.	15
Picallili Beets	1 aver. svg.	60
Pickles—		
Dill or Sour	1 large	15
Sweet	1 small	25
Vinegar	—	0

SUGAR

Brown	1 tsp.	15
Granulated	1 tsp.	18
Maple Sugar	1 tsp.	18
Powdered	1 tsp.	15

| All Spices | — | 0 |

SOUPS & BROTHS

Barley Soup	1 cup	125
Bean Soup	1 cup	200
Beef Broth	1 cup	35
Beef Bouillon	1 cup	30
Beef Consomme	1 cup	35
Beef Soup	1 cup	100
Borscht	1 cup	75
Bouillabaise	1 serving	525
Celery Soup (Clear)	1 cup	100
Chicken Soup	1 cup	75
Chicken Bouillon	1 cup	25
Chicken Broth	1 cup	35
Chicken Gumbo	1 cup	125
Clam Chowder	1 cup	80
Creamed Soups—		
Asparagus	1 cup	200
Celery	1 cup	200
Mushroom	1 cup	200
Oyster	1 cup	200
Pea	1 cup	275
Potato	1 cup	300
Tomato	1 cup	150
Duck Soup	1 cup	125
Minestrone	1 aver. svg.	100
Mock Turtle Soup	1 cup	125
Noodle Soup	1 cup	120
Scotch Broth	1 cup	100
Split Pea Soup	1 cup	150
Tomato Soup (Clear)	1 cup	50
Vegetable Soup	1 cup	85
Vichysoisse	1 cup	275
Won Ton Soup	1 cup	250

SWEETS
Candies, Nuts & T.V. Snacks

Almonds	12–15	100
Almond Chocolate Bar	1	260

Almond Fudge	1″ square	110
Black Walnuts	11 halves	100
Bonbons	1	50
Brazil Nuts	1	25
Brown Sugar Fudge	1″ Square	100
Butter Nuts	5	100
Butterscotch Candy	1 wafer	75
Candied Fruit Peel	1 oz.	100
Caramel	1 aver.	50
Caramel Chocolate Nuts	1 piece	90
Caramel Walnuts	1 piece	50
Cashews	7	75
Chestnuts	8	50
Chewing Gum	1 stick	6
Chocolate Bar	1 aver.	250
Chocolate Creams	1	75
Chocolate Fudge	1″ square	110
Chocolate Mints	3 small	125
Gum Drops	3 large	100
Halavah	1 oz.	125
Hard Candy	1 oz.	110
Hazel Nuts	10	100
Hickory Nuts	8	50
Indian Nuts	1 tbsp.	25
Jelly Beans	15	100
Kisses	1 aver.	40
Lemon Drops	7	100
Lichi Nuts	6	50
Licorice Stick	1 oz.	100
Marshmallows	1	25
Mints (After Dinner)	3 small	125
Orange Drops	2	30
Peanut Brittle	1″ x 2″	50
Peanuts	10	100
Peanut Butter	1 tbsp.	100
Pecans	3	50
Pistachios	16	50
Pizza	½ of 12″ diam.	250
Popcorn (Plain)	1 cup	50
Popcorn (Buttered)	1 cup	150
Pretzels	5 thin sticks	20
	6 aver. sticks	100
Taffy	1″ cube	40
Walnuts	4	100

Almond Cake	1 aver. piece	250
Almond Cookies	2 medium	50
Almond Macaroons	1 large	100
Angel Food Cake	2″ Wedge	100
Animal Cookies	6	50
Anise Cookies	3 small	50
Apple Cake	1 aver. piece	250
Apple Pie	1 aver. piece	275
Apple Pie—Deep Dish	1 aver. piece	325
Apple Pie—French	1 aver. piece	300
Applesauce Cake	1 aver. piece	420
Apricot Pie	1 aver. piece	250
Banana Cake	1 aver. piece	200
Banana Cream Pie	1 aver. piece	350
Blackberry Pie	1 aver. piece	350
Blueberry Cake	1 aver. piece	175
Blueberry Upside-Down Cake	1 aver. piece	275
Blueberry Cream Pie	1 aver. piece	400
Blueberry Pie (Plain)	1 aver. piece	375
Boston Cream Pie	1 aver. piece	400
Boysenberry Pie	1 aver. piece	350
Bridge Cake	1 aver. piece	250
Butter Cookies	6	100
Caramel Cake	1 aver. piece	250
Cheese Cake	1 aver. piece	350
Cherry Upside-Down Cake	1 aver. piece	275
Cherry Pie	1 aver. piece	350
Chocolate Cake	1 aver. piece	250
Chocolate Cookies	3 small	65
Chocolate Cream Pie	1 aver. piece	400
Cinnamon Cake	1 aver. piece	150
Coconut Cake	1 aver. piece	350
Coconut Macaroon	1 large	100
Coconut Cream Pie	1 aver. piece	450
Coconut Custard Pie	1 aver. piece	400
Crumb Cake	2″ x 4″ piece	100
Cupcakes	1 aver.	150
Date Cookies	2 aver.	100
Devil's Food Cake	1 aver. piece	275
Egg Nog Cake	1 aver. piece	175
Elderberry Pie	1 aver piece	350
Fig Bar	1	50
Fruit Cake	½″ Wedge	200

Gingerbread Cake	2″ square	175
Gingersnaps	5	100
Graham Crackers	3 medium	75
Honey Cake	1 aver. piece	100
Huckleberry Pie	1 aver. piece	350
Ice Box Cake	1 aver. piece	300
Ice Box Cookies	3 medium	100
Ladyfinger Cookies	4	100
Lemon Chiffon Pie	1 aver. piece	375
Lemon Cream Pie	1 aver. piece	350
Lemon Meringue Pie	1 aver. piece	350
Lime Chiffon Pie	1 aver. piece	350
Loganberry Pie	1 aver. piece	350
Marble Cake	1 aver. piece	125
Mince Pie	1 aver. piece	350
Oatmeal Cookies	1 large	100
Peach Pie	1 aver. piece	250
Petit Fours	1 aver. piece	100
Pineapple Cream Pie	1 aver. piece	400
Pineapple Pie (Plain)	1 aver. piece	350
Pineapple Upside-Down Cake	1 aver. piece	250
Pound Cake	1 aver. piece	125
Pumpkin Pie	1 aver. piece	325
Raisin Cookies	1 large	50
Raisin Pie	1 aver. piece	400
Raspberry Pie	1 aver. piece	350
Rhubarb Pie	1 aver. piece	400
Sponge Cake	1 aver. piece	125
Strawberry Pie	1 aver. piece	375
Strawberry Cream Pie	1 aver. piece	400
Strawberry Chiffon Pie	1 aver. piece	275
Vanilla Wafers	1 aver.	25
Walnut Cookies	1 large	100
White Cake	1 aver. piece	200

MISCELLANEOUS DESSERTS & SWEETS

Apple Brown Betty	½ cup	200
Apple Cobbler	1 cup	90
Apple Mousse	1 aver. svg.	325
Apple Pudding	½ cup	200
Apple Struedel	1 aver. svg.	225
Apple, Taffy	1	260
Apple Tapioca	½ cup	150
Apple Tart	1 medium	175

Apple Turnover	1 medium	250
Apricot Mousse	1 aver. svg.	350
Apricot Whip	1 aver. svg.	110
Baked Alaska	1 aver. svg.	350
Banana Custard	1 aver. svg.	200
Banana Mousse	1 aver. svg.	350
Banana Split	1	450
Blintz, Cheese	1	175
Blintz, Jelly	1	175
Blueberry Tart	1	225
Bread Pudding	½ cup	125
Brownies	2″ square	150
Butterscotch Pudding	½ cup	175
Cherry Cobbler	1 aver. svg.	300
Chocolate Pudding	½ cup	200
Cinnamon Bun	1	100
Creampuff	1	175
Crullers	1	150
Custard (Plain)	½ cup	125
Danish Pastry (Plain)	1	200
Danish Pastry (Cheese)	1	250
Danish Pastry (Fruit)	1	250
Date Pudding	1 aver. svg.	100
Doughnuts—		
French	1	200
Jelly	1	250
Plain	1	150
Sugar	1	175
Eclair	1	275
Gelatin Dessert	1 aver. svg.	100
Honey	1 tbsp.	65
Ices (All Flavors)	1 aver.	100
Jams & Jellies	1 tbsp.	50
Junket	1 aver. svg.	100
Lemon Whip	1 aver. svg.	40
Marmalade	1 tbsp.	50
Marshmallow	1 aver.	25
Orange Ambrosia	1 aver. svg.	140
Peach Cobbler	1 aver. svg.	300
Peach Mousse	1 aver. svg.	350
Plum Pudding	1 aver. svg.	225
Prune Struedel	1 aver. svg.	225
Prune Whip	1 cup	100
Rice Pudding	½ cup	100
Sherbert (All Flavors)	1 aver. svg.	100

Strawberry Mousse	1 aver. svg.	250
Strawberry Shortcake	1 aver. svg.	250
Strawberry Tart	1	300
Sundaes (All Flavors)	1 aver.	400
Tapioca Pudding	½ cup	140
Turnovers	1 medium	250

Vegetables

Artichoke	1 large	75
Asparagus	1 stalk	3
Avocado	1 medium	400
Bamboo Shoots	1 cup	60
Beans—		
Baked	1 cup	300
Kidney	1 cup	200
Green	1 cup	40
Lima	1 cup	200
Navy	1 cup	200
Yellow	1 cup	40
Bean Sprouts	1 cup	25
Beet Greens	1 cup	40
Beets	1 cup	70
Broccoli	1 cup	40
Brussels Sprouts	1 cup	60
Cabbage—		
Boiled	1 cup	40
Cole Slaw	½ cup	50
Sauerkraut	1 cup	40
Carrots, Cooked	1 cup	40
Carrots, Raw	1 medium	20
Cauliflower	1 cup	30
Celery, Cooked	1 cup	25
Celery, Raw	2 stalks	10
Chard, Cooked	1 cup	50
Collards	1 cup	80
Corn, Canned	1 cup	150
Corn, Fresh	1 medium ear	100
Cucumbers	1 large	25
Dandelion Greens	1 cup	80
Eggplant—	1 cup	50
Italian Style (Baked)	1 aver. svg.	450
Parmigian	1 aver. svg.	600
Scalloped	1 aver. svg.	250
Endive	2 large leaves	10
Escarole	½ heart	10

110

Kale	1 cup	50
Leeks	1 aver. piece	7
Lettuce	¼ head	10
Mushrooms	½ cup	15
Mustard Greens	1 cup	30
Okra	10 pods	30
Onions	1 large	50
Paprika	Sprinkle	1
Parsley (Chopped)	1 tbsp.	2
Parsnips	1 cup	90
Peas	1 cup	100
Pepper, Green	1 large	25
Pepper, Red	1 medium	40
Pimientos	1 aver.	15
Potatoes—		
Baked	1 medium	100
Boiled	1 medium	80
Chips	10 medium	100
French Fried	20 pieces	400
Hash Brown	½ cup	250
Mashed (Milk & Butter)	½ cup	125
Mashed (Plain)	½ cup	75
Sweet Potato	1 small	150
Pumpkin	1 cup	85
Radishes	5	10
Rutabaga	½ cup	30
Sauerkraut	½ cup	30
Scallions	2	10
Spinach	½ cup	25
Squash—		
Acorn	½ cup	50
Butternut	½ cup	18
Hubbard	½ cup	50
Summer	½ cup	18
Winter	½ cup	50
Succotash	½ cup	75
Tomato—		
Fresh	1 medium	25
Juice	½ cup	25
Cooked	1 cup	50
Turnips	1 cup	50
Turnip Greens	1 cup	50
Watercress	1 cup	10
Yams, Baked	1 small	150
Yams, Candied	1 medium	325

The following listing is divided into three groups—according to Brand Name. Although each of these major—and highly representative—manufacturers of frozen foods make a number of other frozen products, this listing is restricted to their *complete frozen dinners* as an aid in totalling calories without having to add up individual parts. The calorie count has been determined by the manufacturers themselves and rounded off by the author within 10 calories.

Note: Simply comparing calories between similar products made by two different manufacturers is not necessarily helpful—as weights and sizes of portions may vary considerably.

BANQUET FROZEN FOODS
(Calorie Count Per Complete Dinner)

Chopped Beef	390
Italian Style	410
Haddock	420
Turkey	280
Beef	300
Salisbury Steak	340
Macaroni & Cheese	340
Mexican Style	570
Ham	350
Beef Enchilada	470
Beans & Franks	690
Fried Chicken	540
Ocean Perch	470
Spaghetti & Meatballs	420
Cheese Enchilada	480
Meat Loaf	420

CHUN KING FROZEN DINNERS
(Calorie Count Per Complete Dinner)

Chicken Chop Suey Dinner	350
Shrimp Chop Suey Dinner	290
Egg Foo Yung Dinner	410
Vegetable Chow Mein Dinner	200
Chicken Chow Mein Dinner	230
Shrimp Chow Mein Dinner	190

Swanson "TV" Dinners
(Calorie Count Per Complete Dinner)

Beans & Franks	610
Beef	410
Chili Con Carne	460
Chopped Sirloin Beef	450
Corned Beef Hash	510
Fried Chicken	600
Fish 'n French Fries	430
Filet of Haddock	400
Ham	370
Loin of Pork	460
Macaroni and Beef	300
Macaroni and Cheese	370
Meat Loaf	420
Noodles and Chicken	370
Fried Shrimp	360
Spaghetti & Meatballs	320
Swiss Steak	360
Turkey	400

"TV" Brand Dinners—International

Chinese Style	360
German Style	410
Italian Style	450
Mexican Style	660

Three Course Dinners

Beef	600
Fried Chicken	650
Salisbury Steak	520
Turkey	560

113

The nutritional "musts" that appear on this page are those usually recommended by nutritionists and dietitians so that you will be able to achieve your full component of daily needs *without the aid of vitamin pills, specialized commercial foods, etc.* The list presumes that you are an adult in good health.

You should therefore get in the habit (if you aren't already) of consuming each of these foods *on your eating day*. With the habit established during the diet itself, you'll have no trouble continuing it at the diet's conclusion.

As to your diet day . . . you *should,* for the most part, attempt to consume each of these foods *or their equivalent.* Commercial preparations (such as Metrecal, Sego, etc.) will indeed act as a viable substitute for these foods—at one meal, two meals or all three meals. A multiple vitamin-with-iron pill will also eliminate the need for *some* of them. In addition, please bear in mind that there is a certain amount of "overlap" from day to day. Eating well on Thursday and Saturday (two eating days) is quite likely to overcome whatever deficiencies may have been present in Friday's diet. Most nutritionists agree that even an occasional day *of complete fast* (should you be so inclined) will not hurt you a bit, provided that your regular eating habits are good.

Having filled your basic requirements, you may then choose more foods *either from this list or not*—in order to meet your particular day's calorie quota:

Milk (or its equivalent in milk products): one pint.

Lean meat, poultry or fish: one small serving (3 ounces).

Eggs: ½ egg will do. (So will 3 or 4 a week.)

Butter or Margarine: 2 tablespoons. (You'll often get this much just in cooking.)

Vegetables (2 servings): leafy, green or yellow.

Fruits (2 servings): Include citrus or tomato.

Bread or Cereal (whole grain or enriched): 2 ounces (equal to two slices).

THE EATING MAN'S DIET MENUS

Important Note
900-Calorie Menus
    900-A
    900-B
    900-C
    For Those Who Enjoy Late Snacks
    Another Late Snack Suggestion
Special 600-Calorie Menu
1600-Calorie Menus
    The Basic Diet
    If You Like to Break Between Meals . . .
    Heavy Date This Evening?
    Movies Tonight!
    How About Some Pizza?
1750-Calorie Menus
    The Basic Diet
    With Snacks
    Bowling Tonight
2000-Calorie Menus
    The Basic Diet
    A Snacker's Delight
    How About a Big, Big Breakfast?
2300-Calorie Menus
    The Basic Diet
    You Say You're Actually Dieting?
2700-Calorie Menus
    The Basic Diet
    If All You Need Is a Couple of Breaks . . .
3000-Calorie Menus
    My Own Basic Diet
    For the In-Between Mealers
3500-Calories
    The Basic Diet

IMPORTANT:
A NOTE ON THESE MENUS

Please be careful as you page through these menus (particularly should you decide to exactly copy any of them yourself) not to "read in" any details which are not actually listed. A broiled veal cutlet, for instance, is 125 calories—but a broiled veal cutlet with a tablespoon of mustard is 135 calories. If you'd prefer a tablespoon of ketchup, the total climbs to 150 calories!

This does not mean we're opposed to condiments. You're welcome to use any and all you'd like—but keep track of them (at least mentally) as you go.

One special thing to watch is the use of butter (or margarine). Often these menus will specifically list its use (with potatoes and other vegetables, bread, etc.). Where it is *not* listed, it is *not* used. At 50 calories per patty, just applying it in an unaccounted-for quantity for twice a day can put an extra pound on you every month.

You'll note, of course, that the emphasis here is on the lower calorie menus—with five 1600-calorie suggestions, only two 2300's and only one 3500. Obviously the more calories that are available to you on an eating day—the easier it is to set your own menu up. Read the lower calorie menus thoroughly no matter how many more calories you may be allowed and I think you'll find they provide a good skeletal construction for you to base menus of your own on.

For the sake of simplicity, *all menus here* (even the 3500-calorie one) contain skimmed milk rather than whole (except where specifically listed) and black coffee rather than with cream and sugar. If you *must* drink whole milk and creamed coffee—fine. Just be sure to take the extra calories into account.

Finally, you will not find any menus here which are EXTRA-ORDINARILY heavy on sweets or other so-called "empty calorie" foods. The purpose of listing these menus is to suggest meals that are both nutritionally and esthetically satisfying with the accent on simple, well-known and easy-to-prepare foods. As the preceding paragraph implies, however, there's nothing really wrong with working from a day's menu somewhat below your actual caloric needs and, having thus assured yourself that your *other* nutritional requirements are fulfilled, stocking up on "empty calories" to meet your quota.

Whatever you do, keep in mind that these menus are no more than mere suggestions and you should adapt them to your own likes and needs.

A SMATTERING OF 900-CALORIE MENUS

It's perfectly true that no matter how you slice, boil, broil or roast 900 calories—they remain, nonetheless, 900 calories. Should you wish to make variations of your own on these menus, be very careful to keep the nutritional "musts" of the previous section in mind.

900 CALORIES—A

Breakfast	Calorie Count
½ grapefruit	50
1 cup dry cereal w/artificial sweetener	110
1 glass skimmed milk (use some of the milk for the cereal)	90
1 hardboiled egg	80
Coffee, black (w/artificial sweetener; drink as much as you'd like)	0
Total:	330

Lunch	
½ cup chicken chow mein	125
¾ cup boiled white rice w/one pat of margarine	150
Two cups tea w/lemon	6
1 small apple	50
Total:	331

Supper	
Lettuce and tomato salad with low calorie dressing (one tablespoon)	42
6 boiled shrimp	60
1 slice protein bread w/margarine	100
1 large tangerine	35
2 glasses diet ginger ale	2
Total:	239
Daily Total:	900

900 CALORIES—B

Breakfast	
¼ honeydew melon	65
1 cup dry cereal w/artificial sweetener	110
1 glass skimmed milk (use some of the milk for the cereal)	90

Coffee, black (w/artificial sweetener; drink as much
as you'd like)	0
Total:	265

Lunch

1 cup chicken bouillon	25
Fried egg sandwich (1 egg fried without fat; 2 slices protein bread; 1 pat margarine)	230
1 medium peach	50
Tea, black (w/artificial sweetener)	0
Total:	305

Supper

⅛ lettuce head w/1 tbsp. low calorie dressing	17
Skimmed milk	90
Baked red snapper	100
½ cup cole slaw	50
3 olives	25
2 stalks celery	10
½ medium orange	37
Total:	329
Daily Total:	899

900 Calories—C

Breakfast

1 cup dry cereal w/artificial sweetener	110
1 glass skimmed milk (use some of the milk for the cereal)	90
½ banana (slice into the cereal)	50
Coffee, black (w/artificial sweetener; drink as much as you'd like)	0
Total:	250

Lunch

1 cup tomato soup	50
2 Ry-Krisp	35
1 poached egg	80
1 cup plain yogurt, mixed with ¼ cup of blackberries	175
2 glasses diet cola	2
Total:	342

Supper

1 small steak	150
1 slice protein bread w/margarine	100
½ cup peas	50
2 cups tea w/lemon	6
Total:	306
Daily Total:	898

900 CALORIES—D
FOR THOSE WHO ENJOY LATE SNACKS

Breakfast

4 oz. tomato juice	25
2 slices protein bread, toasted, w/margarine (2)	200
Coffee, black (w/artificial sweetener)	0
Total:	225

Lunch

1 broiled veal cutlet	125
½ cup spinach	25
1 glass skimmed milk	90
Total:	240

Supper

1 cup vegetable soup	85
¼ cup oyster crackers	30
1 hard boiled egg	80
1 small orange	50
Tea, black (w/artificial sweetener)	0
Total:	245

Late Snack

1 glass skimmed milk	90
1 banana	100
Total:	190
Daily Total:	900

900 CALORIES—E
ANOTHER LATE SNACK SUGGESTION

Breakfast

1 cup hot oatmeal w/artificial sweetener	150
1 glass skimmed milk (use some of the milk for the oatmeal)	90
Coffee, black (w/artificial sweetener)	0
Total:	240

Lunch

Clam chowder	80
1 zweiback toast w/margarine	80
1 sliced cucumber	25
½ cup fresh strawberries w/artificial sweetener	25
Tea, black (w/artificial sweetener)	0
Total:	210

Supper

1 slice pork loin roast	100
¼ cup canned pineapple	100
5 radishes	10
1 slice protein bread w/margarine	100
Total:	310

Late Snack

1 glass skimmed milk	90
2 vanilla wafers	50
Total:	140
Daily Total:	900

SPECIAL 600 CALORIE MENU

Feel like really cutting down today? Try this special 600-calorie menu. All your nutritional "musts" are well represented.

Breakfast

½ grapefruit	50
1 slice protein toast w/margarine	100
1 glass skimmed milk	90
Coffee, black (w/artificial sweetener)	0
Total:	240

Lunch

1 slice protein bread w/margarine	100
2 scallions	10
1 glass skimmed milk	90
1 plum	30
1 glass diet cola	1
Total:	231

Supper

⅛ head of lettuce w/1 tbsp. low calorie dressing	17
1 cup beef bouillon	30

6 oysters on the halfshell	50
½ cup summer squash	18
5 radishes	10
Black coffee w/ artificial sweetener	0
Total:	125

Before Bed

2 glasses diet ginger ale	2
Daily Total:	598

1600 CALORIES
THE BASIC DIET

Breakfast

4 oz. tomato juice	25
¼ honeydew melon	65
Dry cereal w/1 tsp. sugar	128
1 glass skimmed milk (use some on your cereal)	90
1 slice cinnamon toast (protein bread w/1 pat margarine, 1 tsp. sugar mixed with cinnamon)	118
Coffee, black (w/ artificial sweetener)	0
Total:	426

Lunch

1 cup chicken soup	75
Meat Loaf (aver. svg.)	225
Baked potato w/ margarine	150
½ cup spinach	25
1 medium slice watermelon	100
Tea, black (w/ artificial sweetener)	0
Total:	575

Supper

Lettuce and tomato salad w/1 tbsp. low calorie dressing	42
Chicken a la king	375
1 glass skimmed milk	90
Apple cobbler	90
Total:	597
Daily Total:	1599

If You Like to Break Between Meals . . .

Breakfast

½ grapefruit	50
1 cup dry cereal w/artificial sweetener	110
1 glass skimmed milk (use some of this milk on your cereal)	90
1 hardboiled egg	80
Coffee, black (w/artificial sweetener)	0
Total:	330

Coffee Break

1 sugar doughnut	175
Coffee, black	0
Total:	175

Lunch

Veal stew (aver. svg.)	250
1 whole wheat bread w/margarine	125
Gelatin dessert	100
Total:	475

Afternoon Break

3 small chocolate cookies	65
Tea w/lemon	3
Total:	68

Supper

Lettuce and tomato salad w/low calorie dressing	42
Baked chicken (aver. svg.)	200
1 slice whole wheat bread w/margarine	125
1 glass skimmed milk	90
½ cup green beans	20
Total:	477

Late Snack

One medium apple	75
1 glass diet cola	1
Total:	76
Daily Total:	1598

Remember, it isn't recommended that you defer your heavier eating until late in the day—as a matter of course. Even 90-pounders like yourself enjoy really tying on the feedbag once in awhile though—especially at a fine restaurant—and especially if your guy is glad to pay for it. You can have a dandy meal with no guilty conscience if you'll pay attention to *the entire day's* calories.

Breakfast

½ grapefruit		50
Poached egg		80
1 slice protein bread w/margarine		100
Black coffee w/artificial sweetener		0
	Total:	230

Lunch

¼ cantaloupe		25
1 cup beef broth		35
2 Ry-Krisp		35
3 radishes		6
1 diet cola		1
	Total:	102

Supper

Martini w/olive		135
1 cup Scotch broth w/croutons		125
Lettuce and tomato salad w/2 tbsp. Roquefort dressing		100
Filet mignon (aver. svg.)		250
1 medium baked potato w/sour cream		200
½ cup rutabaga w/butter		80
1 small roll w/butter		125
Lime ice w/2 vanilla cookies		150
1 cup tea w/lemon		3
Blackberry cordial		100
	Total:	1268
	Daily Total:	1600

Breakfast

½ grapefruit	50
1 cup dry cereal w/1 tsp. sugar	28
1 glass skimmed milk (use some on the cereal)	90
Black coffee (w/artificial sweetener)	0
Total:	268

Coffee Break

1 Cinnamon Roll	100
Black coffee	0
Total:	100

Lunch

1 cup cream of oyster soup	200
3 Ry-Krisp	50
Fried egg on rye (fried without fat; 2 slices rye bread; 1 tbsp. mayonnaise)	350
1 glass diet gingerale	1
Total:	601

Afternoon Break

1 medium apple	75

Supper

1 cup chicken broth	25
Chicken giblets (aver. svg.)	150
½ cup carrots w/margarine	70
1 stalk celery	5
2 cups tea, black w/lemon	6
Total:	256

At The Movies

1 cup buttered popcorn (buy a full box—about 2 cups—and share with date)	150

After The Show

16 pistachios	50
1 glass of beer (8 oz.)	100
Evening's Total:	300
Daily Total:	1600

1600 CALORIES
HOW ABOUT SOME PIZZA?

Breakfast

½ grapefruit	50
1 poached egg	80
1 slice protein toast w/margarine	100
1 glass skimmed milk	90
Coffee, black (w/artificial sweetener)	0
Total:	320

Lunch

1 cup chicken bouillon	25
1 sandwich (2 slices cracked wheat bread, 2 slices bologna, 1 slice Swiss cheese, 1 tbsp. mustard)	400
1 raw carrot	20
1 medium orange	75
2 cups black tea w/lemon	6
Total:	526

Supper

1 lettuce and tomato salad w/1 tbsp. low calorie dressing	42
6 medium deviled clams	100
½ cup boiled cabbage	20
1 glass skimmed milk	90
1 small apple	50
Total:	302

At The Pizza Parlor

½ small (12″ diameter) pizza—plain or with mushrooms	250
2 glasses of beer (8 oz. each)	200
Total:	450
Daily Total:	1598

1750 CALORIES
THE BASIC DIET

Breakfast

4 oz. tomato juice	25
½ grapefruit	50
1 cup dry cereal w/1 tsp. sugar	128
1 glass skimmed milk (use some on cereal)	90

1 softboiled egg	80
1 slice whole wheat toast w/margarine	125
Coffee, black (w/artificial sweetener)	0
Total:	498

Lunch

1 cup clam chowder	80
1 onion roll w/margarine	200
Barbecued spare ribs (6)	250
½ cup lima beans	100
Gelatin dessert	100
1 cup tea w/lemon	3
Total:	733

Supper

Lettuce and tomato salad w/1 tbsp. low calorie dressing	42
1 aver. svg. of liver	150
½ cup brussels sprouts	30
1 boiled potato w/butter	130
1 glass skimmed milk	90
3 almond cookies	75
Total:	517
Daily Total:	1748

1750 CALORIES
WITH SNACKS

Breakfast

Tomato juice (4 oz.)	25
½ grapefruit	50
2 softboiled eggs	160
1 slice protein bread w/ma. 'arine	100
1 glass skimmed milk	90
Coffee, black (w/artificial sweetener)	0
Total:	425

Coffee Break

1 plain doughnut	150
Coffee, black	0
Total:	150

Lunch

Lettuce and tomato salad w/1 tbsp. low calorie dressing	42
1 cup beef stew	250
1 slice cracked wheat bread w/margarine	110
Gelatin dessert	100
1 glass diet gingerale	1
Total:	502

Afternoon Break

2 fig bars	100
1 glass skimmed milk	90
Total:	190

Supper

½ cup chicken bouillon	12
2 slices fried ham	200
Potatoes mashed w/milk and butter	125
½ cup sauerkraut	20
Tea, black (w/artificial sweetener)	0
Total:	357

Evening Snack

Marble cake (1 aver. piece)	125
Sanka	0
Total:	125
Daily Total:	1749

1750 CALORIES
BOWLING TONIGHT

Breakfast

1 cup oatmeal w/1 pat margarine and 1 tsp. sugar	218
1 glass skimmed milk (use some on cereal)	90
3 oz. fresh orange juice	37
Coffee, black (w/artificial sweetener)	0
Total:	345

Lunch

Beef broth	35
Bacon, lettuce & tomato on toast (3 slices bacon, 1 or 2 lettuce leaves, ½ sliced tomato, 1 tbsp. mayonnaise, 2 slices white bread)	384

1 medium apple tart		175
Tea, black (w/artificial sweetener)		0
	Total:	594

Supper

1 broiled pork chop		225
½ cup cabbage		20
1 slice protein bread w/margarine		100
1 glass skimmed milk		90
	Total:	435

At The Lanes

3 glasses of beer (8 oz. each)		300
4 aver. pretzels		75
	Total:	375
	Daily Total:	1749

2000 CALORIES
THE BASIC DIET

Breakfast

3 oz. fresh orange juice		35
2 slices of french toast w/2 pats of margarine and 2 tbsp. maple syrup		470
Coffee, black (w/artificial sweetener)		0
	Total:	505

Lunch

Tomato and lettuce salad w/2 tbsp. low calorie dressing		54
1 beef pot pie		450
3 saltine crackers w/1 pat margarine		95
1 glass skimmed milk		90
1 aver. svg. strawberry shortcake		250
	Total:	929

Supper

1 cup noodle soup		120
2 slices pork loin roast		200
¼ cup canned pineapple		100
½ cup beets		35
1 slice vienna bread w/margarine		110
Tea, black (w/artificial sweetener)		0
	Total:	565
	Daily Total:	1999

2000 CALORIES
A SNACKER'S DELIGHT

Breakfast

½ grapefruit	50
2 pancakes w/2 pats margarine and 2 tbsp. maple syrup	380
2 strips lean bacon	80
Coffee, black (w/artificial sweetener)	0
Total:	510

Coffee Break

1 cheese blintz	175
Coffee, black	0
Total:	175

Lunch

1 cup chicken chow mein	250
1 cup Chinese fried rice	200
1 scoop ice cream	150
Tea, black (w/artificial sweetener)	0
Total:	600

Afternoon Break

1 extra large tomato w/salt	50

Supper

1 cup chicken bouillon	25
1 knockwurst sausage on hard roll	350
½ cup acorn squash w/margarine	100
1 glass skimmed milk	90
Total:	565

Just Before Bed

1 banana	100
Daily Total:	2000

2000 CALORIES
HOW ABOUT A BIG, BIG BREAKFAST?

Breakfast

1 glass tomato juice (4 oz.)	25
½ grapefruit	50
2 slices cracked wheat toast w/2 pats of margarine and 2 tbsp. strawberry jam	320

2 eggs fried without fat	160
3 strips lean bacon	120
1 cup dry cereal w/1 tsp. sugar	128
1 glass skimmed milk (use some on cereal)	90
Coffee, black (w/artificial sweetener)	0
Total:	893

Lunch

Broiled halibut (aver. svg.)	200
1 tbsp. tartar sauce	100
½ cup yellow beans w/margarine	70
10 potato chips	100
1 glass skimmed milk	90
1 svg. lemon whip	40
Total:	600

Supper

Shrimp cocktail (5 shrimp, 1 tbsp. cocktail sauce)	100
1 aver. svg. roast turkey	175
2 tbsp. cranberry sauce	67
2 stalks celery	10
1 corn muffin w/margarine	150
1 cup black tea w/lemon	3
Total:	505
Daily Total:	1998

2300 CALORIES
THE BASIC DIET

Breakfast

Tomato juice	25
½ grapefruit	50
1 buckwheat waffle w/2 pats of margarine and 2 tbsp. maple syrup	445
2 sausage links	150
Coffee, black (w/artificial sweetener)	0
Total:	670

Lunch

1 cup tomato soup	50
3 saltine crackers	45
1 svg. barbecued beef	300
½ cup acorn squash w/margarine	100
½ cup peas w/butter	100

Parkerhouse roll w/butter	150
1 aver. piece crumb cake (2″ x 4″)	100
1 cup black tea w/lemon	3
Total:	848

Supper

12 french fried shrimp	240
1 svg. hash brown potatoes w/1 pat margarine	300
½ cup cole slaw	50
1 glass skimmed milk	90
½ cup fruit cocktail	100
Total:	780
Daily Total:	2298

2300 CALORIES
YOU SAY YOU'RE ACTUALLY DIETING?

Breakfast

½ cantaloupe	50
1 cup dry cereal w/1 tsp. sugar	128
1 glass skimmed milk (use some on cereal)	90
2 slices raisin toast w/2 pats margarine	270
Coffee, black (w/artificial sweetener)	0
Total:	538

Coffee Break

1 cheese danish	250
Coffee, black	0
Total:	250

Lunch

1 cup vegetable soup	85
1 medium steak "smothered in mushrooms"	240
1 medium baked potato w/margarine	150
⅔ cup corn w/margarine	150
1 glass diet cola	1
Total:	626

Afternoon Break

1 large orange	100

Supper

Tomato and lettuce salad w/1 tbsp. low calorie dressing	42

Roast pheasant		175
½ cup acorn squash w/margarine		100
½ cup green beans w/margarine		70
1 slice rye bread w/margarine		135
1 cup black tea w/lemon		3
1 aver. piece angel food cake		100
	Total:	625

Before Bed

6 potato chips		60
1 glass of ale (8 oz.)		100
	Total:	160
	Daily Total:	2299

2700 Calories
The Basic Diet

With this many calories to consume on your eating day, a generous breakfast becomes a must. Enjoy it.

Breakfast

½ grapefruit		50
Tomato juice		25
2 eggs fried without fat		160
1 small steak		150
1 cup dry cereal w/1 tsp. sugar		128
1 glass skimmed milk		90
2 slices white toast w/2 pats margarine and 2 tbsp. honey		380
Coffee, black (w/artificial sweetener)		0
	Total:	983

Lunch

1 cup vegetable soup		85
2 lamb chops		400
1 svg. potatoes mashed w/milk and butter		125
½ cup peas w/margarine		100
1 glass skimmed milk		90
1 aver. svg. tapioca pudding		140
	Total:	940

Supper

| Lobster cocktail | | 90 |
| Tomato and lettuce salad w/1 tbsp. low calorie dressing | | 42 |

Aver. svg. chicken a la king		375
½ cup green beans w/butter		70
1 glass skimmed milk		90
	Total:	667

Nightcap

| 1 whiskey and soda | | 100 |
| | Daily Total: | 2690 |

2700 CALORIES
IF ALL YOU NEED IS A COUPLE OF BREAKS . . .

Breakfast

6 oz. orange juice		75
1 cup dry cereal w/1 tsp. sugar		128
1 glass skimmed milk (use some on sugar)		90
2 boiled eggs		160
2 white toast w/2 pats margarine		270
Coffee, black (w/artificial sweetener)		0
	Total:	723

Coffee Break

1 sugar doughnut		175
Coffee, black		0
	Total:	175

Lunch

Tomato and lettuce salad w/1 tbsp. low calorie dressing		42
Scallops (6, fried)		400
French fries (20 pieces)		400
1 glass skimmed milk		90
1 apple tart		175
	Total:	1107

Supper

1 aver. svg. beef liver		150
1 small yam w/margarine		200
¾ cup sauerkraut		30
1 caraway roll w/margarine		175
Tea, black (w/artificial sweetener)		0
	Total:	555

133

Nightcap:

1 glass dry sauterne	75
8 almonds	65
Total:	140
Daily Total:	2700

3000 CALORIES
MY OWN BASIC DIET

Remember this one from the Introduction? It's highly representative of my eating days throughout six months of the diet and, as you'll note, I go just a little over in this case—although it's easily seen the few extra calories may be eliminated by having only one Scotch before retiring instead of two—or even cutting out a single pat of butter somewhere during the day.

Breakfast

½ grapefruit	50
4 oz. tomato juice	25
1 cup dry cereal w/1 tsp. sugar	128
1 glass skimmed milk (a little on the cereal)	90
1 slice fried ham	100
Double egg omelet (fried without fat) w/1 tbsp. provolone cheese and 1 tbsp. jelly	245
½ parboiled potato fried without fat	40
2 protein toast w/2 pats margarine and 2 tbsp. honey	330
Coffee, black (w/artificial sweetener)	0
Total:	1008

Lunch

Tomato and lettuce salad—no dressing	30
1 cup clam chowder (called a "bowl" in restaurants)	80
2 small rolls w/2 butter	250
1 small steak	150
1 baked potato w/butter	150
½ cup stringbeans	20
Deep dish apple pie a la mode	475
Coffee, black	0
Total:	1155

Supper

Martini w/olive	135
Tomato and lettuce salad w/low calorie dressing (1 tbsp.)	42

Chicken bouillon	25
1 aver. svg. baked chicken	200
½ cup broccoli	20
Potatoes mashed w/milk and margarine	125
1 piece rye bread w/margarine	135
1 cup tea w/lemon	3
Total:	685

Nightcap

| 2 Scotch and sodas | 200 |
| Daily Total: | 3048 |

3000 CALORIES
FOR THE IN-BETWEEN MEALERS

Breakfast

½ grapefruit	50
4 oz. tomato juice	25
3 pancakes w/2 pats margarine and 2 tbsp. maple syrup	470
2 slices fried ham	200
Coffee, black (w/artificial sweetener)	0
Total:	745

Coffee Break

1 fruit danish	250
Coffee, black	0
Total:	250

Lunch

1 cup chicken broth	25
Tomato and lettuce salad w/1 tbsp. low calorie dressing	42
Beef stroganoff (aver. svg.)	350
1 Parkerhouse roll w/margarine	150
2 scoops ice cream	300
1 cup black tea w/lemon	3
Total:	870

Afternoon Break

1 cup of blackberries	100
4 oz. whole milk	85
2 tsp. sugar	35
Total:	220

Broiled whitefish (aver. svg.)		125
1 svg. french fries (20)		400
½ cup brussels sprouts w/margarine		80
1 slice rye bread w/margarine		135
Coffee, black		0
	Total:	740

Late Snack

1 apple tart		175
1 Sanka, black		0
	Total:	175
	Daily Total:	3000

3500 CALORIES
THE BASIC DIET

There is such a wide latitude in a 3500-calorie diet—both in variety and quantity of food—that some may wonder why we bother to list even a single day's sample menu. The reason, of course, is that a man whose ideal weight is 200 pounds has to eat *so very much* each day just to keep from losing weight that it may seem to him that there is no true limit on his calorie count . . . which is nonsense.

You'll note that the Basic Diet described here—listing only one in-between meals' snack—not only depends on the use of black coffee, artificial sweetener and skimmed milk, but allows double portions only once (2 pork chops at supper) and has no provision for dessert after that meal. Naturally the 3500-calorie consumer *can* adjust his eating day meals so that he's allowed creamed coffee, sugar, whole milk, more than one double portion and perhaps even an extra dessert and a nightcap. The point is, however—just as in the case of the 90-pound, 1600-calorie consumer—he has no choice but to *make such changes with caution.*

Breakfast

6 oz. tomato juice	35
½ grapefruit	50
2 eggs (fried without fat)	160
1 small steak	150
1 cup dry cereal w/2 tsp. sugar	145
1 glass skimmed milk (use some on cereal)	90

2 slices white toast w/2 pats margarine and 2 tbsp. honey	370
Coffee, black (w/artificial sweetener)	0
Total:	1000

Coffee Break

1 sugar doughnut	175
Coffee, black	0
Total:	175

Lunch

1 tomato and lettuce salad w/1 tbsp. low calorie dressing	42
1 cup split pea soup	200
3 soda crackers	25
Chicken fricassee (aver. svg.)	225
½ cup peas w/margarine	100
2 slices garlic bread w/margarine	270
1 piece cherry pie a la mode	500
Tea, black (w/artificial sweetener)	0
Total:	1362

Supper

1 cup chicken soup	75
5 radishes	10
2 scallions	10
2 pork chops	450
1 aver. svg. potatoes mashed w/milk and margarine —add 1 extra pat margarine	175
½ cup lima beans w/margarine	150
1 glass skimmed milk	90
Total:	960
Daily Total:	3497

Name _____ Present Weight _____ Ideal Weight _____

Daily Calorie Allowance: Minimum _____ *Diet Ideal* _____ Maximum _____

Date of Beginning _____ Date of Completion _____